Cold & Flu-Busting Recipes for Unwell Days

The Comforting & Nourishing Cookbook

by Olivia Rana

Olivia Rana © 2023

❀❀❀❀❀❀❀❀❀❀❀❀❀❀❀❀❀

License Notes

Table of Contents

Introduction 6

Additional Useful & Interesting Information 8

1. Chicken Noodle Soup with Basil 10

2. Marinated Oranges 13

3. Rosemary Carrots 15

4. Kale & Garlic 17

5. Orange Spiced Carrots 20

6. Chicken Soup with Tomatoes...22

7. Spinach Rice..25

8. Lemon Thyme Green Tea 27

9. Hot Apple Cider 29

10. Carrot Soup with Fennel 31

11. Chicken & Garlic...34

12. Herbed Root Veggies 37

13. Chicken Potpie Soup 40

14. Watercress & Orange Salad 43

15. Mediterranean Chicken Soup 45

16. Orange Salad with Poppy Seeds 48

17. Chicken with Orange Salsa 50

18. Chicken & Turmeric Soup 52

19. Vegetarian Minestrone 55

20. Mixed Green Salad with Orange Vinaigrette 58

21. Pumpkin Bisque 60

22. Carrot Chowder 63

23. Tomato Soup 65

24. Ambrosia Salad 67

25. Vegetable Soup 69

26. Fruit Cup 72

27. Ginger & Kale Smoothie 74

28. Chicken Stir Fry with Honey 76

29. Gingered Brussels Sprouts 79

30. Turkey Minestrone 81

31. Chicken & Vegetable Pasta 84

32. Berry & Yogurt Pops 87

33. Carrot Casserole 89

34. Green Beans with Garlic & Bacon 92

35. Garlic Roasted Vegetables 95

36. Butternut Squash Soup 97

37. Root Vegetable Soup 100

38. Melon & Citrus Medley 103

39. Carrot Soup with Tarragon & Orange 105

40. Honeydew, Strawberry & Cucumber Salad 108

41. Fruit Salad with Honey & Lime Dressing 110

42. Mashed Cauliflower with Garlic 112

43. Candied Carrots 114

44. Ginger, Lemon & Honey Tonic 116

45. Tortellini Soup with Garlic 118

46. Pumpkin Pie Smoothie 120

47. Honey & Cinnamon Rolls 122

48. Lemon Rice Pilaf 125

49. Green Shakshuka 127

50. Spinach with Garlic & Mushrooms 130

Conclusion 132

Biography 133

Afterword 134

Introduction

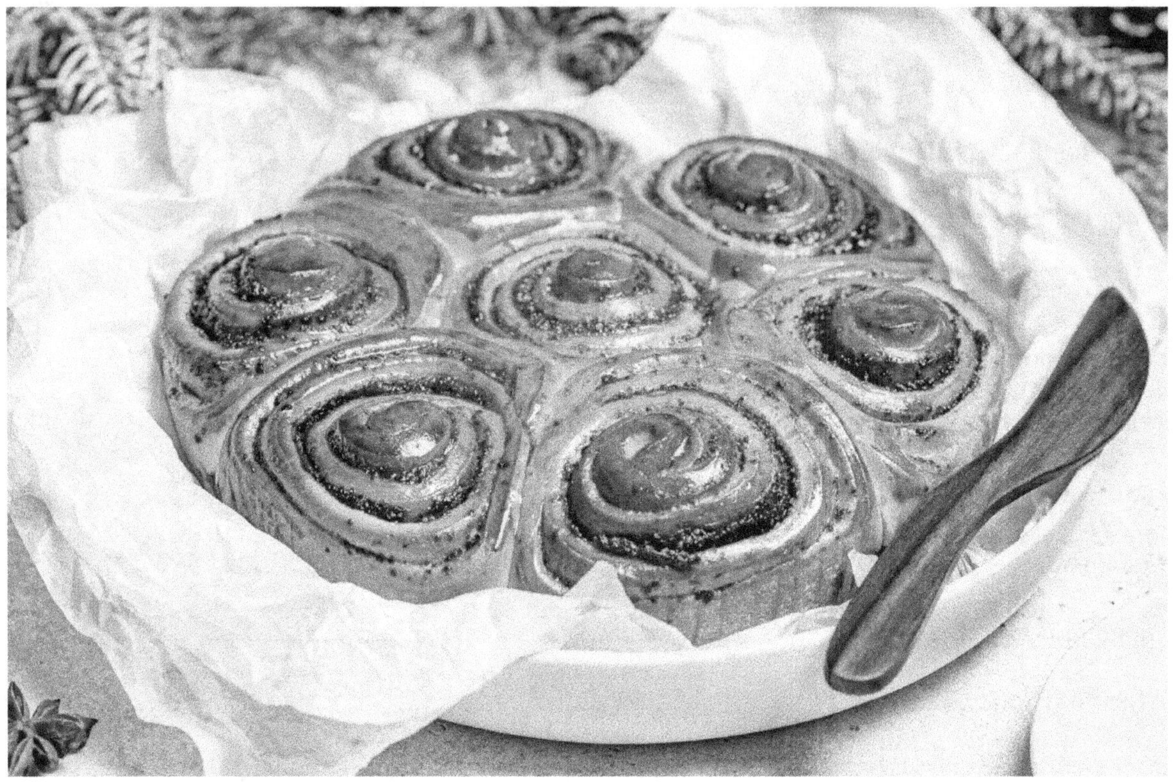

Feeling under the weather?

It may be that time of the year once more when everyone is going down with a cold or flu, and can't seem to get through a whole week without a sneeze or cough.

In this book, you'll find recipes that are not only so delicious that you'd find yourself instantly feeling better, but are also loaded with nourishing vitamins and minerals to strengthen your body's immune defense against illness.

Even if you feel like you don't have the energy to get out of bed, these recipes are simple and easy enough to prepare. Or you can ask your family or friends to prepare something for you.

If things don't get better after a few days, be sure to give your doctor a call, or drop by the clinic for a checkup.

Additional Useful & Interesting Information

To know the difference between cold and flu, here are the signs and symptoms to watch out for.

Signs and symptoms of cold

- Sneezing
- Runny nose
- Nasal congestion
- Sore throat
- Coughing
- Post nasal drip
- Watery eyes

Signs and symptoms of flu

- Fever
- Chills
- Cough
- Sore throat
- Runny nose
- Nasal congestion
- Body aches
- Headache
- Fatigue

Aside from feeding yourself with the right nourishing diet, it's also imperative to get ample rest. Do not engage in activities that will stress you out as this will make your immune defenses weaker.

1. Chicken Noodle Soup with Basil

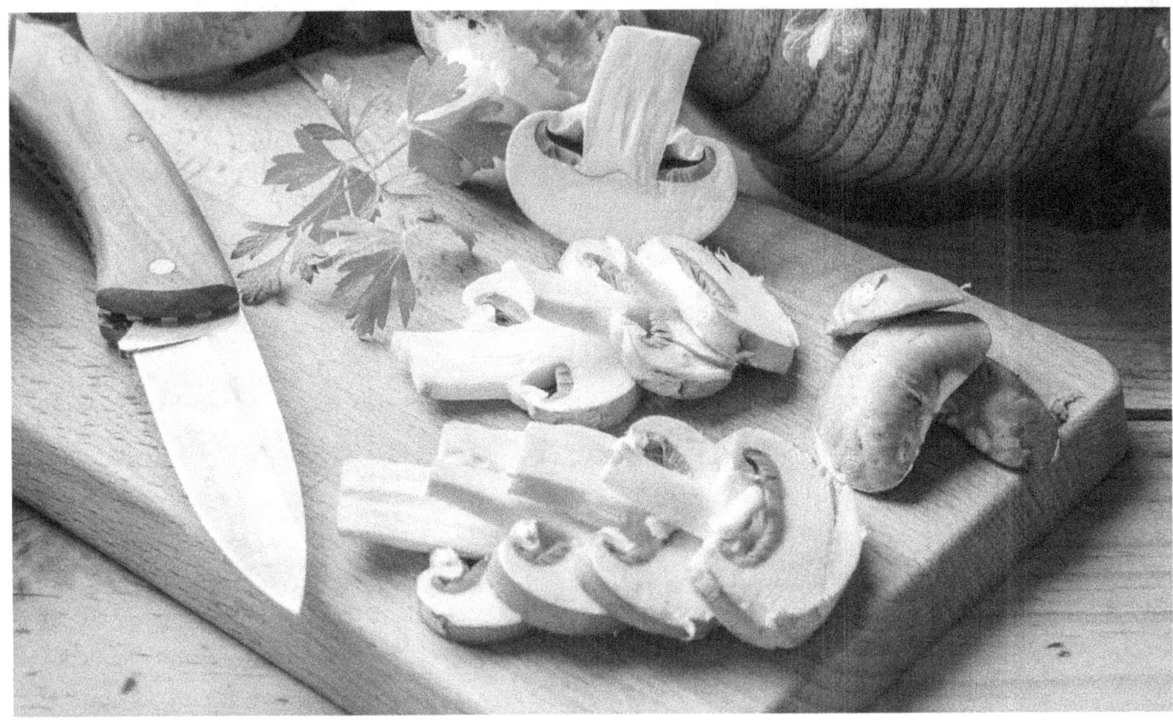

Here's a bowl of nourishing chicken noodle soup to fight off your cold or flu. What makes this version different is the addition of kale and basil, resulting in a dish that's not only more flavorful but also more effective in combating illnesses.

Serving Size: 6

Preparation & Cooking Time: 1 hour and 15 minutes

Ingredients:

- ¼ cup butter, sliced into cubes
- 1 onion, chopped
- ¾ cup mushrooms, chopped
- 2 carrots, chopped
- 2 ribs celery, chopped
- 1 clove garlic, minced
- 64 oz. low sodium chicken broth
- ¼ cup all purpose flour
- 1 ½ teaspoons dried basil
- Pinch salt
- 12 oz. egg noodles
- 2 cups cooked chicken, shredded
- 4 cups fresh kale, chopped

Instructions:

Add the butter to a pot over medium heat.

Cook the onion, mushrooms, carrots and celery for 10 minutes, stirring often.

Stir in the garlic.

Cook for 1 minute.

In a bowl, mix the chicken broth, flour, dried basil and salt.

Pour the mixture into the pot.

Bring to a boil.

Reduce heat and simmer for 10 minutes.

Return to a boil.

Add the egg noodles.

Reduce heat and simmer for 15 minutes.

Add the chicken and kale.

Simmer for 6 minutes until the noodles are tender.

Ladle into soup bowls.

Serve warm.

2. Marinated Oranges

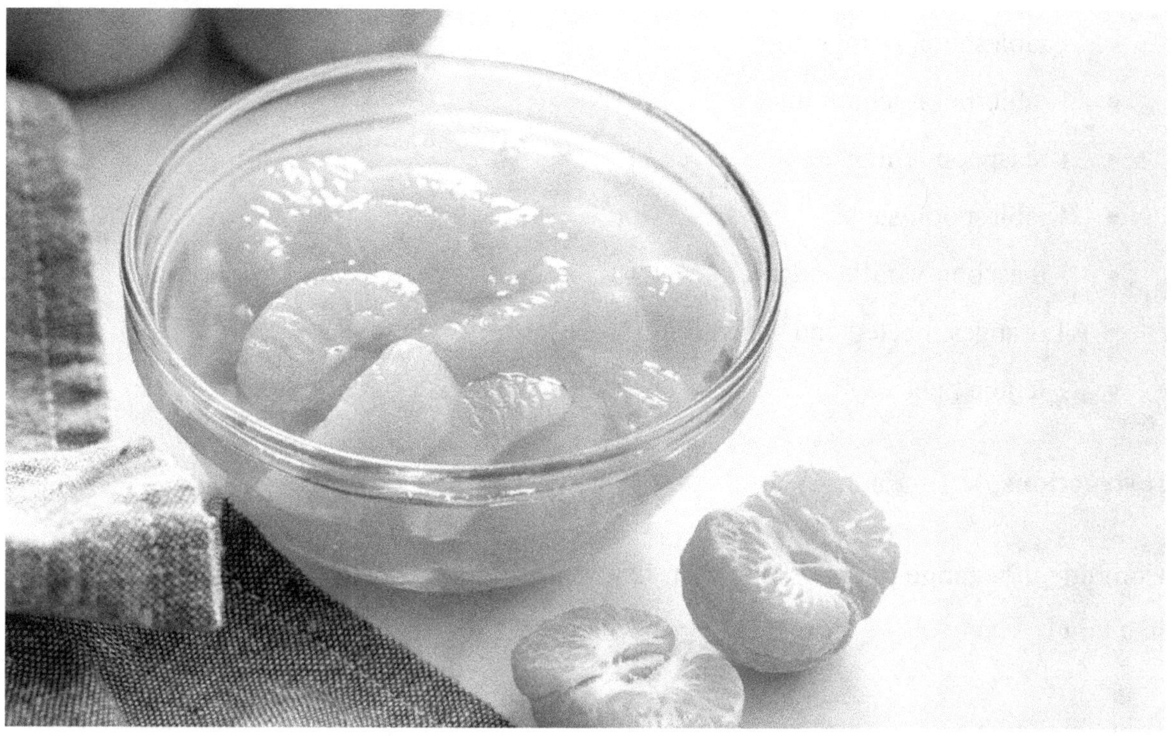

These marinated oranges will not only help treat your cold, but will also cheer you up when you're feeling under the weather.

Serving Size: 4

Preparation & Cooking Time: 2 hours and 15 minutes

Ingredients:

- 1 cup orange juice
- 1 tablespoon orange zest
- 1 tablespoon lemon juice
- 1 teaspoon lemon zest
- 1 tablespoon sugar
- 1 teaspoon vanilla extract
- 4 oranges, peeled and sliced thinly
- 1 lemon peel

Instructions:

Combine the orange juice, orange zest, lemon juice, lemon zest, sugar and vanilla extract in a bowl.

Add the oranges.

Cover and refrigerate for 2 hours.

Top with lemon peel before serving.

3. Rosemary Carrots

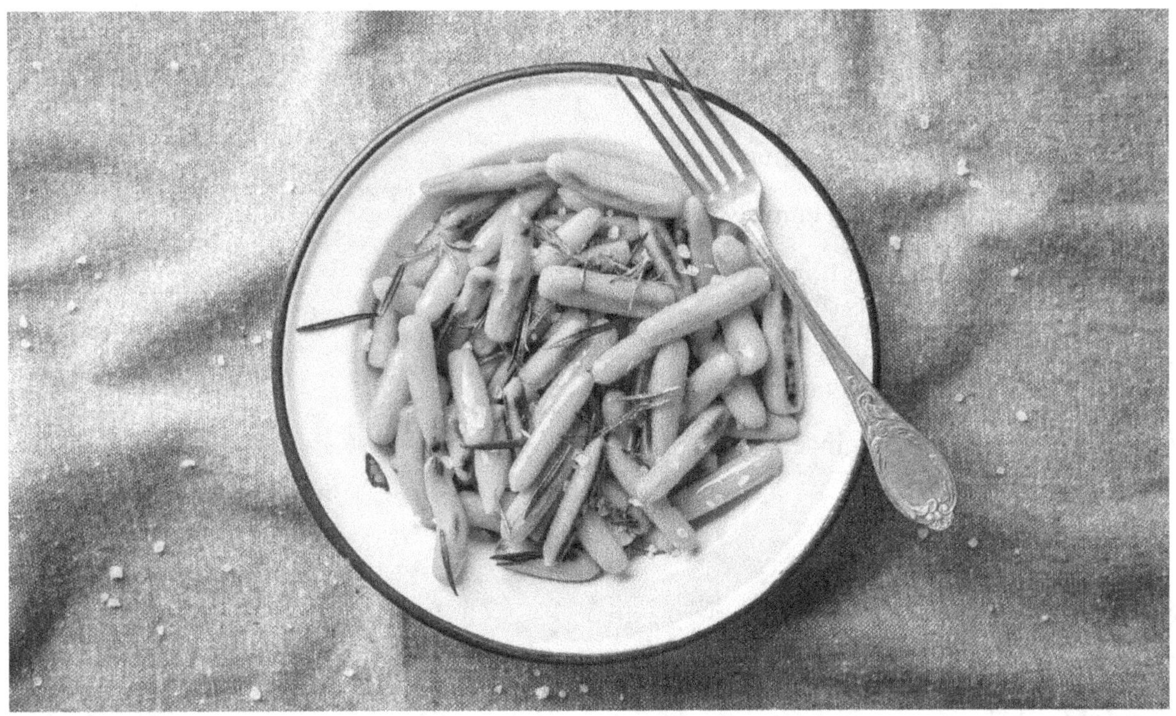

Carrots are full of vitamin C which helps boost immune function. So if you're not feeling well, this recipe is definitely a good idea to prepare. If fresh rosemary is not available, you can also use dried.

Serving Size: 8

Preparation & Cooking Time: 40 minutes

Ingredients:

- 2 lb. baby carrots
- 2 tablespoons olive oil
- 2 cloves garlic, minced
- 2 teaspoons fresh rosemary, minced
- ½ teaspoon ground cumin
- ½ teaspoon onion powder
- 4 teaspoons brown sugar
- Salt and pepper to taste
- 2 green onions, minced

Instructions:

Preheat your oven to 425 degrees F.

Spread the baby carrots in a roasting pan.

In a bowl, combine the olive oil, garlic, rosemary, ground cumin, onion powder, brown sugar, salt and pepper.

Pour the mixture over the carrots.

Toss to mix evenly.

Roast the carrots in the oven for 30 minutes, stirring once.

Sprinkle the green onions on top before serving.

4. Kale & Garlic

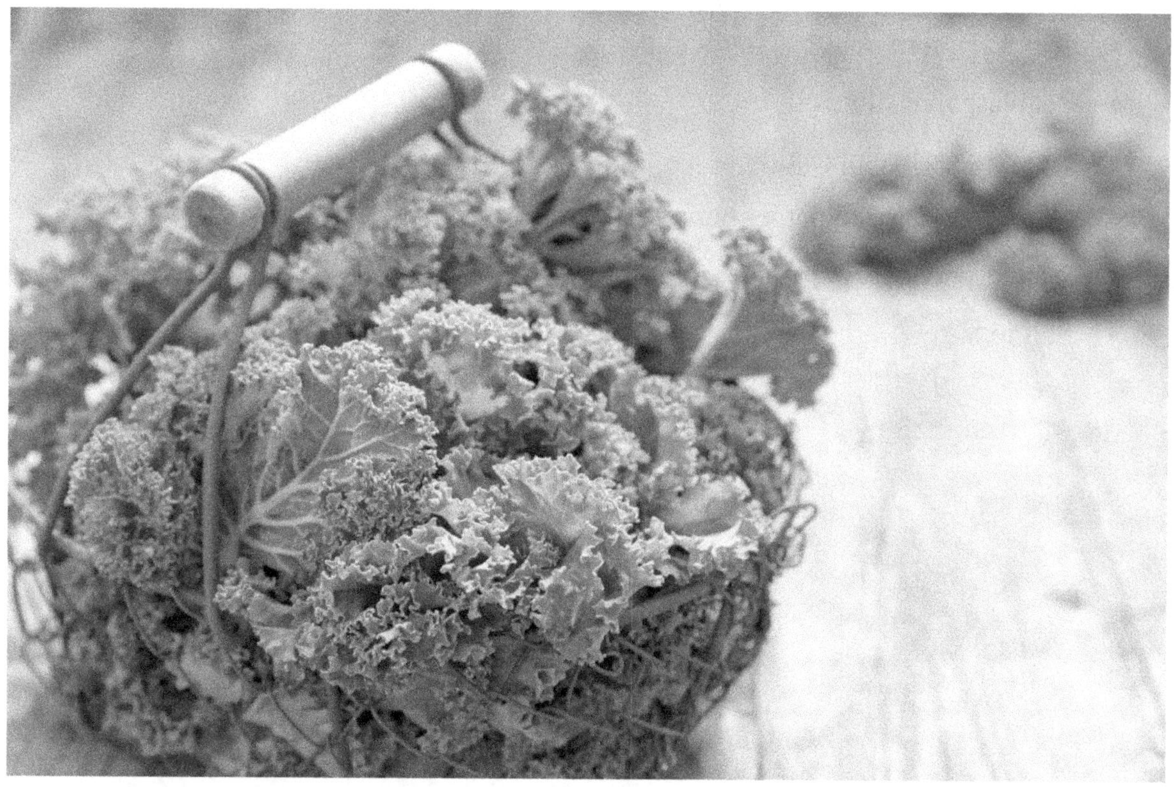

Both kale and garlic are excellent fighters of infections. But of course, you can prepare this dish anytime, and not only when you're feeling unwell.

Serving Size: 4

Preparation & Cooking Time: 30 minutes

Ingredients:

- Water
- 1 lb. kale, torn
- 2 tablespoons olive oil
- 5 cloves garlic, minced
- ¼ cup sun-dried tomatoes chopped
- 2 tablespoons fresh parsley, minced
- Salt to taste

Instructions:

Add 1 inch water to a pot over medium heat.

Bring to a boil.

Add the kale leaves.

Cook while covered for 10 to 15 minutes.

Transfer to a strainer. Discard the liquid.

Pour the olive oil into a pot over medium heat.

Cook the garlic and tomatoes for 1 minute, stirring often.

Add the kale to the pot.

Stir in the parsley.

Season with the salt.

Heat through for 2 to 3 minutes, stirring often.

5. Orange Spiced Carrots

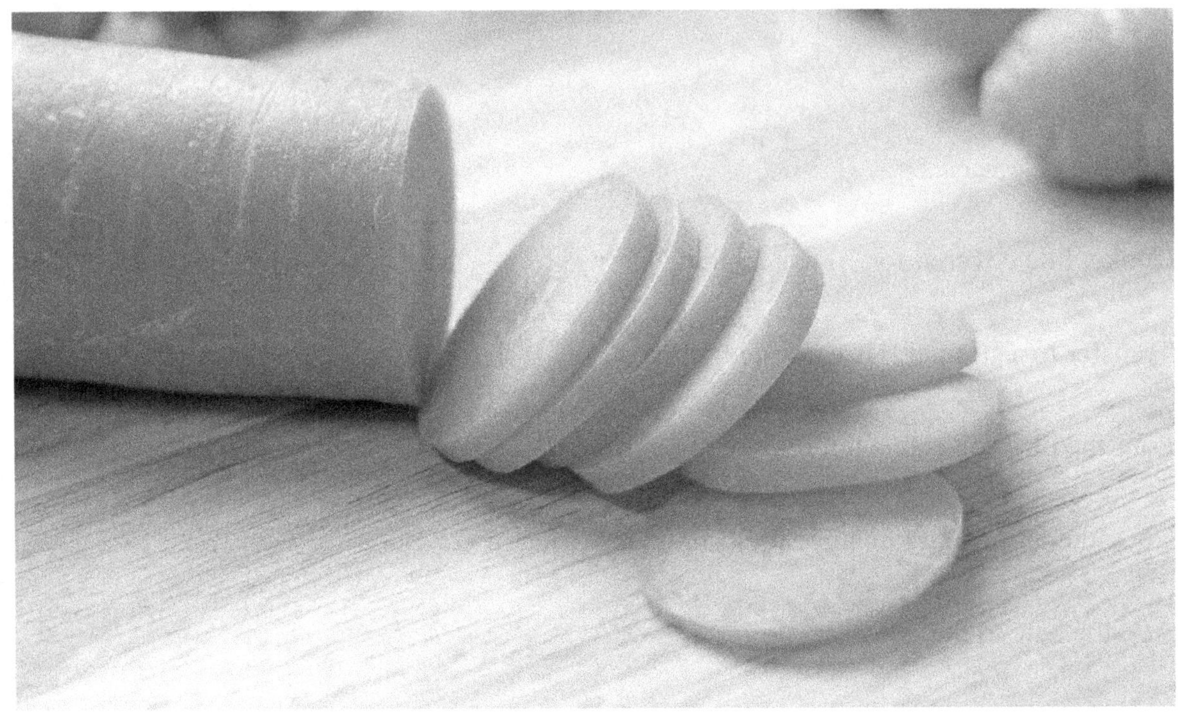

Flavor up your carrots with cinnamon, orange juice and brown sugar for a dish that doesn't only dazzle, but can also help make you feel better.

Serving Size: 6

Preparation & Cooking Time: 4 hours and 10 minutes

Ingredients:

- 2 tablespoons butter
- ½ cup orange juice
- ½ cup brown sugar
- ¼ teaspoon ground nutmeg
- ¾ teaspoon ground cinnamon
- Salt to taste
- 2 lb. carrots, sliced
- 4 teaspoons cornstarch
- ¼ cup cold water

Instructions:

Add the butter, orange juice, brown sugar, ground nutmeg, ground cinnamon and salt in a slow cooker.

Mix well.

Stir in the carrots.

Cover and cook on low for 4 hours.

In a small bowl, mix the cornstarch and water.

Pour the mixture into the carrots.

Cook for 2 minutes or until the sauce has thickened.

6. Chicken Soup with Tomatoes

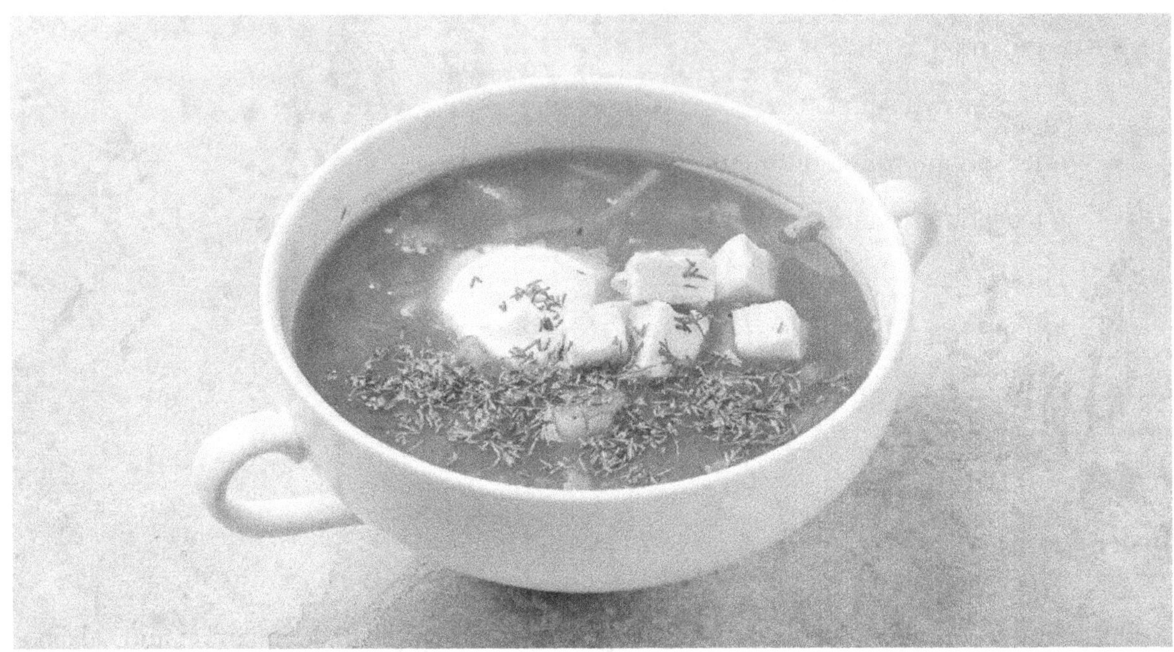

Up the ante of the classic chicken soup with tomatoes, salsa and more vegetables. A bowl of this nourishing soup can help make you feel better in an instant.

Serving Size: 10

Preparation & Cooking Time: 1 hour and 10 minutes

Ingredients:

- 1 ¼ lb. chicken breast fillets
- 4 cups water
- 1 tablespoon canola oil
- 1 onion, chopped
- 4 cloves garlic, minced
- 2 ribs celery, chopped
- 8 oz. tomato sauce
- 28 oz. canned diced tomatoes
- 1 cup salsa
- 2 carrots, sliced
- 3 zucchini, sliced
- 1 cup corn kernels
- 4 oz. green chili, chopped
- 1 teaspoon dried basil
- 2 teaspoons chili powder
- 3 teaspoons ground cumin
- Cheddar cheese, shredded

Instructions:

Add the chicken to a pot over medium heat.

Pour in the water.

Bring to a boil.

Reduce heat and simmer for 15 minutes.

Transfer the chicken to a chopping board.

Slice the chicken into cubes and set aside.

Pour the oil into a pan over medium high heat.

Cook the onion, garlic and celery until tender, stirring often.

Pour in the tomato sauce, canned tomatoes and salsa.

Stir in the carrots, zucchini, corn and green chili.

Season with the dried basil, chili powder and ground cumin.

Bring to a boil.

Reduce heat and simmer for 20 minutes.

Add the chicken to the pot.

Heat through for 5 minutes.

Top with the cheese before serving.

7. Spinach Rice

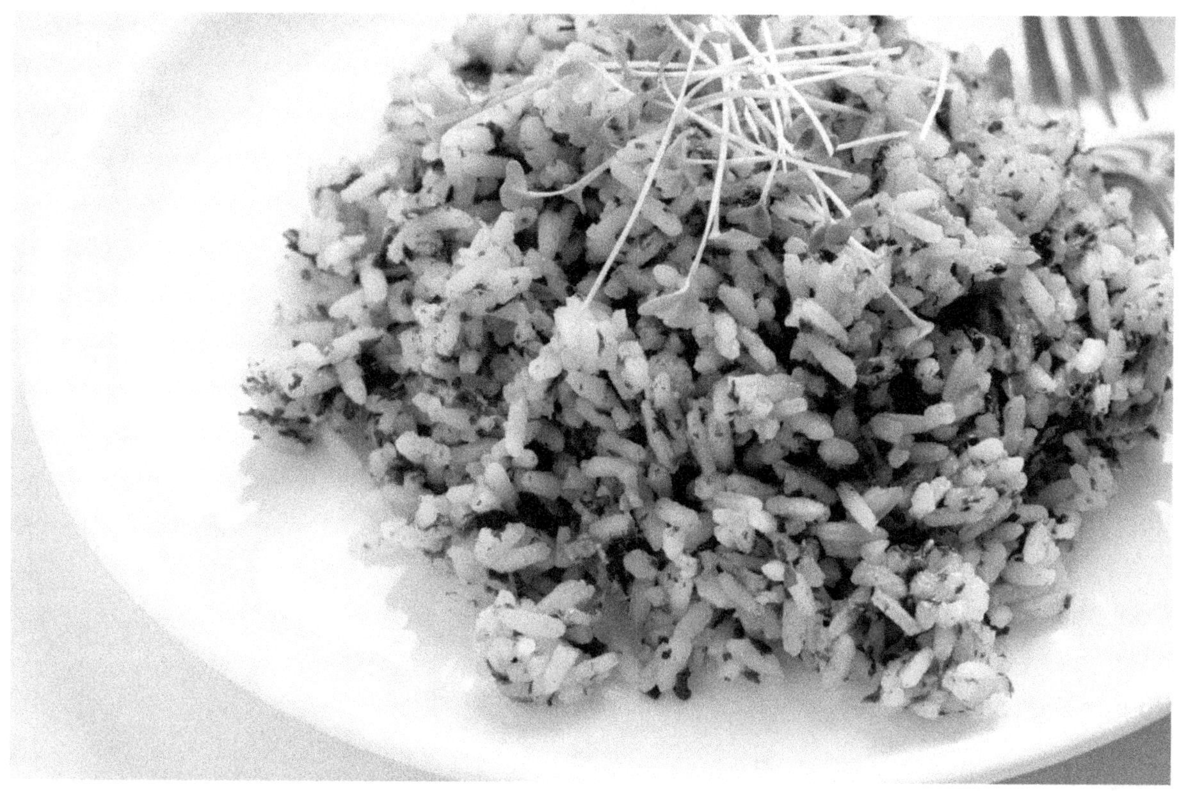

This Greek-inspired dish is something to look forward to when you're not feeling well. Spinach is packed with antioxidants that can boost your immunity. Not to mention, the flavors will inevitably delight you.

Serving Size: 2

Preparation & Cooking Time: 20 minutes

Ingredients:

- 2 tablespoons olive oil
- ½ cup onion, chopped
- ¾ cup water
- 1 tablespoon dried parsley flakes
- Salt and pepper to taste
- ½ cup instant rice (uncooked)
- 2 cups fresh baby spinach

Instructions:

Pour the olive oil into a pan over medium high heat.

Cook the onion until tender.

Pour in the water.

Stir in the parsley.

Season with the salt and pepper.

Bring to a boil.

Add the rice and top with the spinach.

Cover and remove from the stove.

Let sit for 10 minutes until the rice is tender.

Stir before serving.

8. Lemon Thyme Green Tea

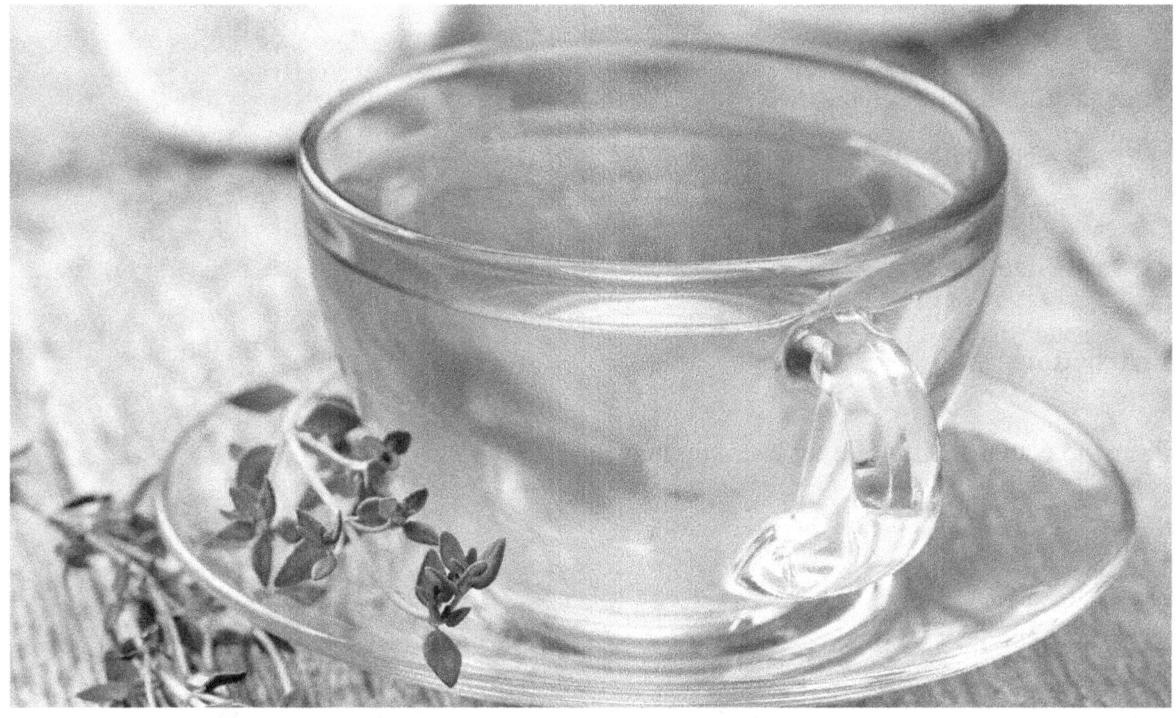

Lemon thyme powers up your cup of green tea to help ward off illnesses.

Serving Size: 8

Preparation & Cooking Time: 20 minutes

Ingredients:

- 2 quarts water
- 8 green tea bags
- ½ teaspoon lemon zest
- 12 sprigs fresh lemon thyme
- 3 tablespoons lemon juice
- ¼ cup honey

Instructions:

Pour the water into a pot over medium heat.

Bring to a boil.

Turn off heat.

Add the tea bags, lemon zest and lemon thyme.

Cover and steep for 3 minutes.

Discard the tea bags.

Steep for 3 more minutes.

Strain the tea.

Stir in the lemon juice and honey.

Serve warm.

9. Hot Apple Cider

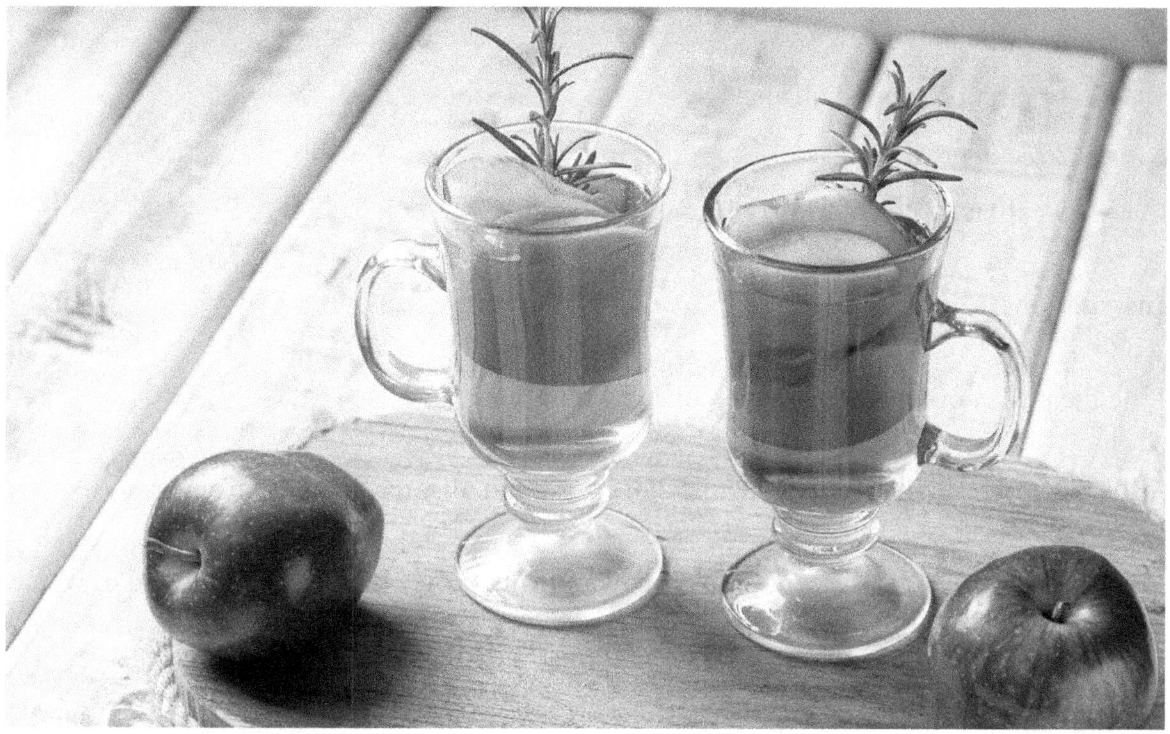

Sugar and spices add extra flavor to warm apple cider.

Serving Size: 20

Preparation & Cooking Time: 15 minutes

Ingredients:

- 3 cinnamon sticks
- 1 teaspoon whole cloves
- 1 teaspoon ground allspice
- 2/3 cup brown sugar
- 1 gallon apple cider

Instructions:

Line the basket of an automatic percolator with a filter.

Fill it up with cinnamon sticks, whole cloves, ground allspice and brown sugar.

Prepare the apple cider the same way you would with coffee but use cider instead of water.

10. Carrot Soup with Fennel

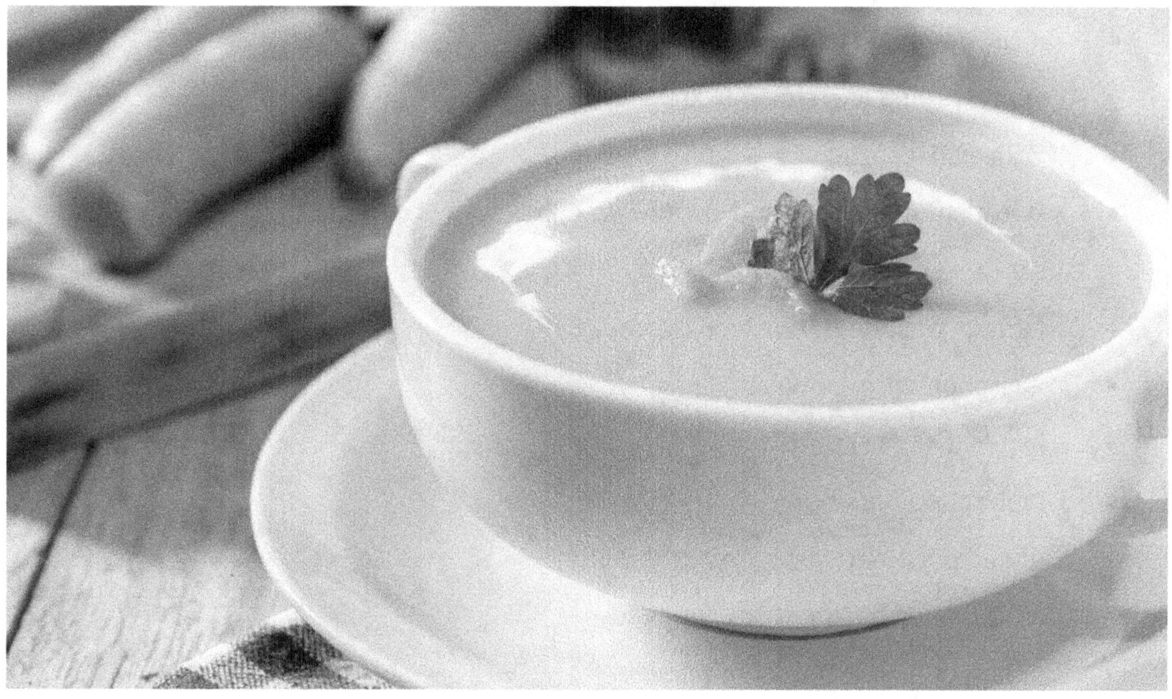

Toasted fennel seeds, carrots, sweet potato and apple combine to create this tasty and creamy soup dish.

Serving Size: 8

Preparation & Cooking Time: 1 hour and 15 minutes

Ingredients:

- 1 tablespoon butter
- ½ teaspoon fennel seed
- 1 apple, peeled and sliced into cubes
- 1 ½ lb. carrots, sliced
- 1 sweet potato, peeled and sliced into cubes
- 43.5 oz. vegetable broth
- 2 tablespoons long grain rice (uncooked)
- ¼ teaspoon curry powder
- 1 bay leaf
- 1 tablespoon lemon juice
- Salt and pepper to taste
- 2 tablespoons fresh parsley, minced
- 2 tablespoons minced fresh parsley

Instructions:

Add the butter to a pan over medium heat.

Cook the fennel for 2 to 3 minutes or until toasted.

Stir in the apple, carrots, and sweet potato.

Cook while stirring for 5 minutes.

Pour in the vegetable broth.

Add the rice, curry powder and bay leaf.

Mix well.

Bring to a boil.

Reduce heat and simmer for 30 minutes or until the rice is tender.

Turn off heat.

Let cool for a few minutes.

Discard the bay leaf.

Puree the mixture in a blender.

Add the pureed mixture back to the pan.

Stir in the lemon juice.

Season with the salt and pepper.

Heat through for 5 minutes.

Top with the parsley before serving.

11. Chicken & Garlic

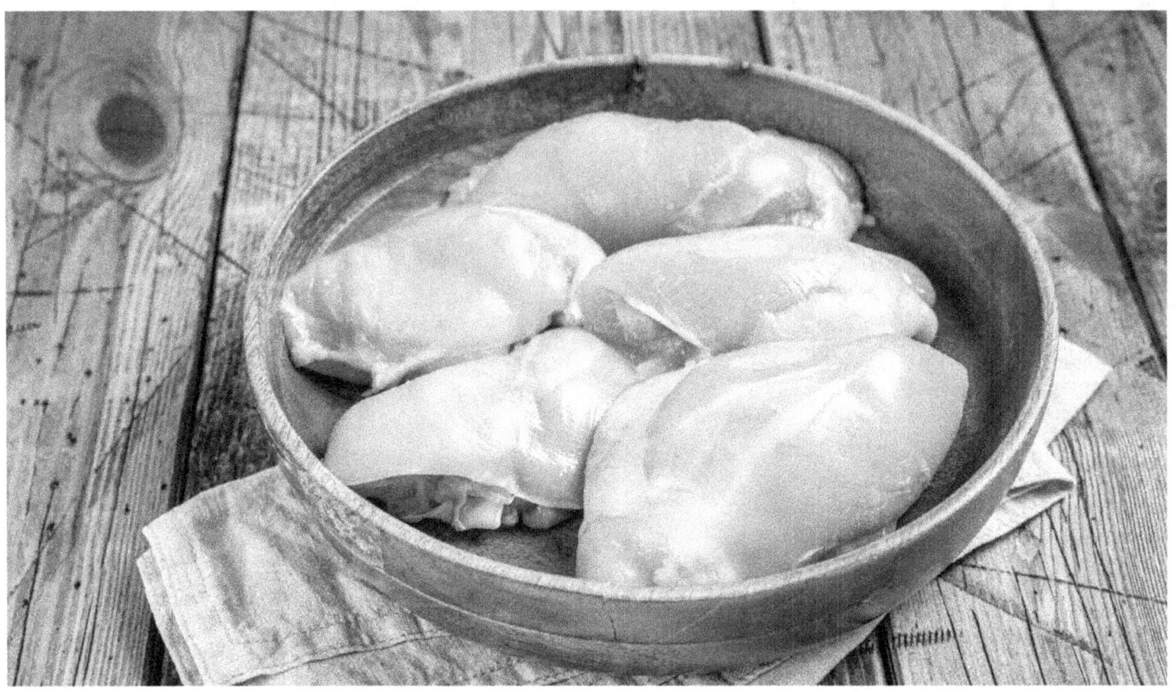

Research has proven that garlic is indeed effective in fighting off infections whether viral or bacterial. So if you're trying to combat an illness, it'd be a great idea to prepare this recipe. Serve this dish with Italian bread or mashed potatoes.

Serving Size: 6

Preparation & Cooking Time: 30 minutes

Ingredients:

- 1 ½ lb. chicken thigh fillets
- Salt and pepper to taste
- 1 tablespoon olive oil
- 10 cloves garlic, peeled and sliced in half
- 1 cup chicken stock
- ½ teaspoon fresh thyme, minced
- 1 teaspoon fresh rosemary, minced
- 1 tablespoon fresh chives, minced

Instructions:

Season the chicken with salt and pepper.

Pour the olive oil into a pan over medium heat.

Cook the chicken until browned on both sides.

Transfer the chicken to a plate.

Next, add the garlic cloves to the pan.

Cook while stirring for 2 minutes.

Pour in the chicken stock and add the herbs.

Return the chicken to the pan.

Bring to a boil.

Reduce heat and simmer for 8 minutes.

12. Herbed Root Veggies

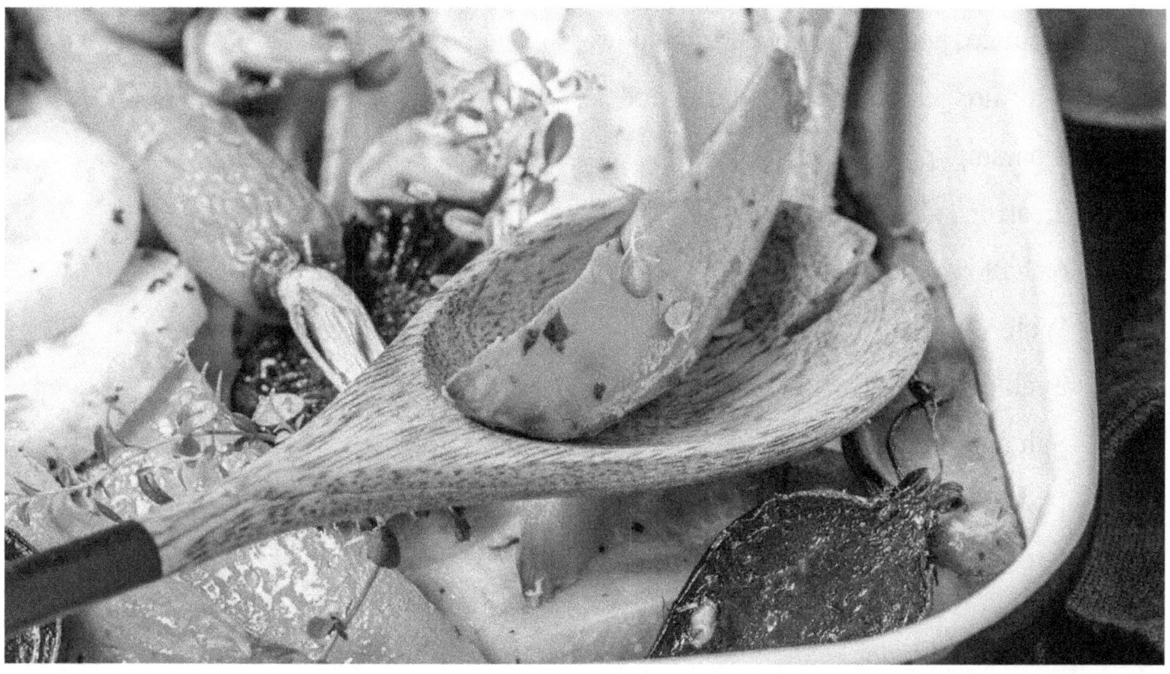

Here's an easy-to -prepare side dish that you can prepare anytime or even when you're not feeling well. It's so easy and won't take so much effort.

Serving Size: 10

Preparation & Cooking Time: 50 minutes

Ingredients:

- 1 sweet potato, peeled and sliced into cubes
- 1 potato, peeled and sliced into cubes
- 1 turnip, peeled and sliced into cubes
- 1 parsnip, peeled and sliced
- 2 carrots, sliced
- 6 shallots, chopped
- Water
- 3 tablespoons olive oil
- Salt and pepper to taste
- 5 to 6 sprigs fresh rosemary
- 5 to 6 sprigs fresh thyme

Instructions:

Preheat your oven to 425 degrees F.

Add the sweet potato, potato, turnip, parsnip, carrots and shallots to pot over medium heat.

Cover with water.

Bring to a boil.

Cover the pot and cook for 7 minutes.

Drain the vegetables and transfer to a bowl.

Toss the vegetables in the olive oil.

Season with the salt and pepper.

Spread the vegetables in a baking pan.

Top with the herb sprigs.

Bake in the oven for 20 minutes, stirring from time to time.

Discard the herb sprigs before serving.

13. Chicken Potpie Soup

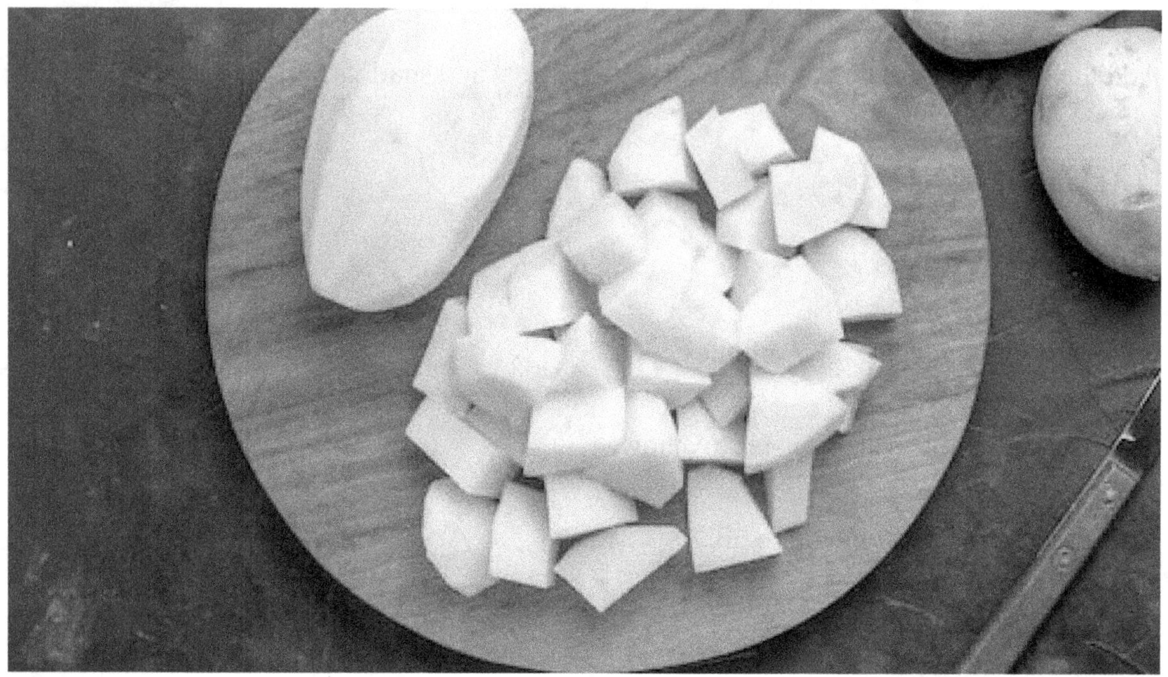

Here's an incredible potpie soup recipe that you'd find yourself craving for even when you're not sick!

Serving Size: 6

Preparation & Cooking Time: 1 hour and 20 minutes

Ingredients:

- 2 cups all purpose flour
- Salt to taste
- 2/3 cup shortening
- 5 tablespoons

Soup

- 2 tablespoons butter
- 1 cup sweet onion, chopped
- 2 ribs celery, chopped
- 1 cup potatoes, peeled and sliced into cubes
- 2 carrots, chopped
- ½ cup all purpose flour
- Salt and pepper to taste
- 43.5 oz. chicken broth
- 2 cups cooked chicken, shredded
- 1 cup peas
- 1 cup corn kernels

Instructions:

Combine the all purpose flour and salt in a bowl.

Stir in the shortening until the texture is crumbly.

Add the milk and knead the dough.

Shape it into a disk.

Cover and refrigerate for 30 minutes.

Preheat your oven to 425 degrees F.

Roll the dough into 1/8 inch thick.

Cut 18 rounds using a round cutter.

Place these in a baking pan.

Bake in the oven for 10 minutes or until golden.

Let cool on a wire rack.

Prepare the soup by adding the butter to a pot over medium high heat.

Cook the onion, celery, potatoes and carrots for 5 minutes or until tender.

Stir in the flour.

Season with the salt and pepper.

Add the broth.

Bring to a boil.

Reduce heat and simmer for 10 minutes.

Add the remaining ingredients.

Ladle into a soup bowl and top with the pie crusts.

14. Watercress & Orange Salad

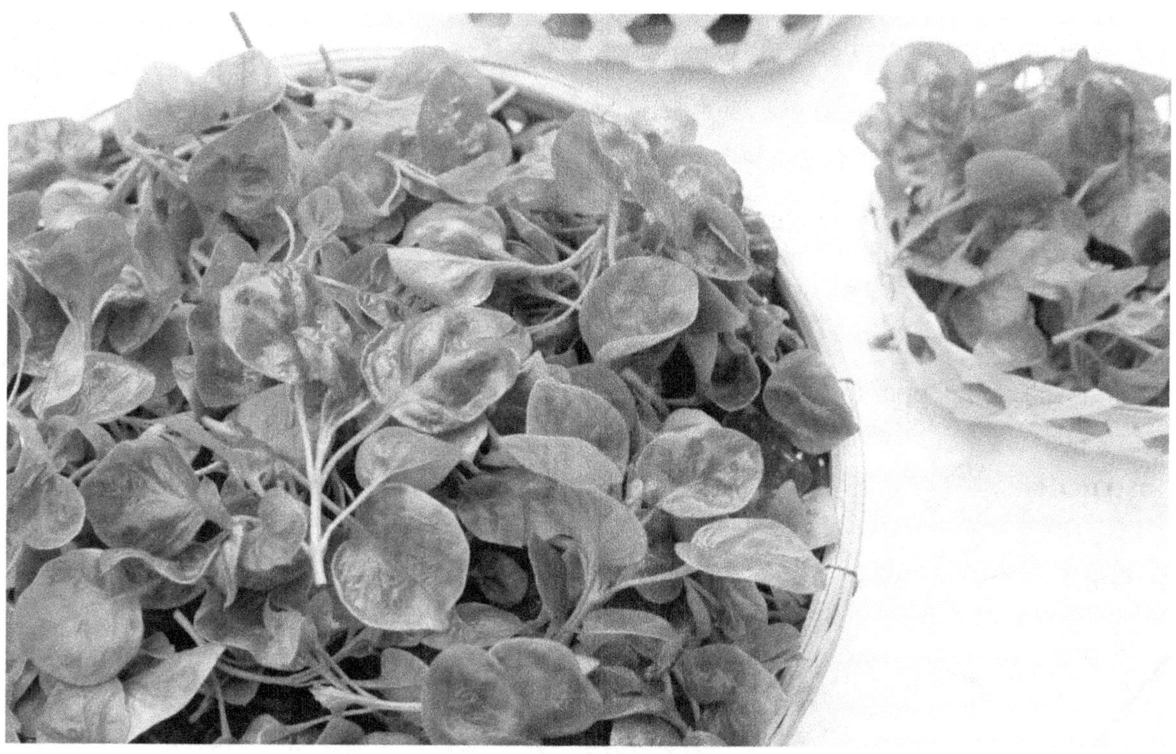

Here's a quick and simple salad recipe that helps boost your immune response to illnesses.

Serving Size: 12

Preparation & Cooking Time: 20 minutes

Ingredients:

- 10 cups watercress, trimmed
- 4 oranges, peeled and sliced
- ¼ cup olive oil
- ½ teaspoon lemon juice
- 3 tablespoons orange juice
- 2 teaspoons orange zest
- ¼ teaspoon sugar
- Salt and pepper to taste

Instructions:

Arrange the watercress in a bowl.

Top with the oranges.

In another bowl, mix the remaining ingredients.

Drizzle the dressing over the salad, toss to combine, and serve.

15. Mediterranean Chicken Soup

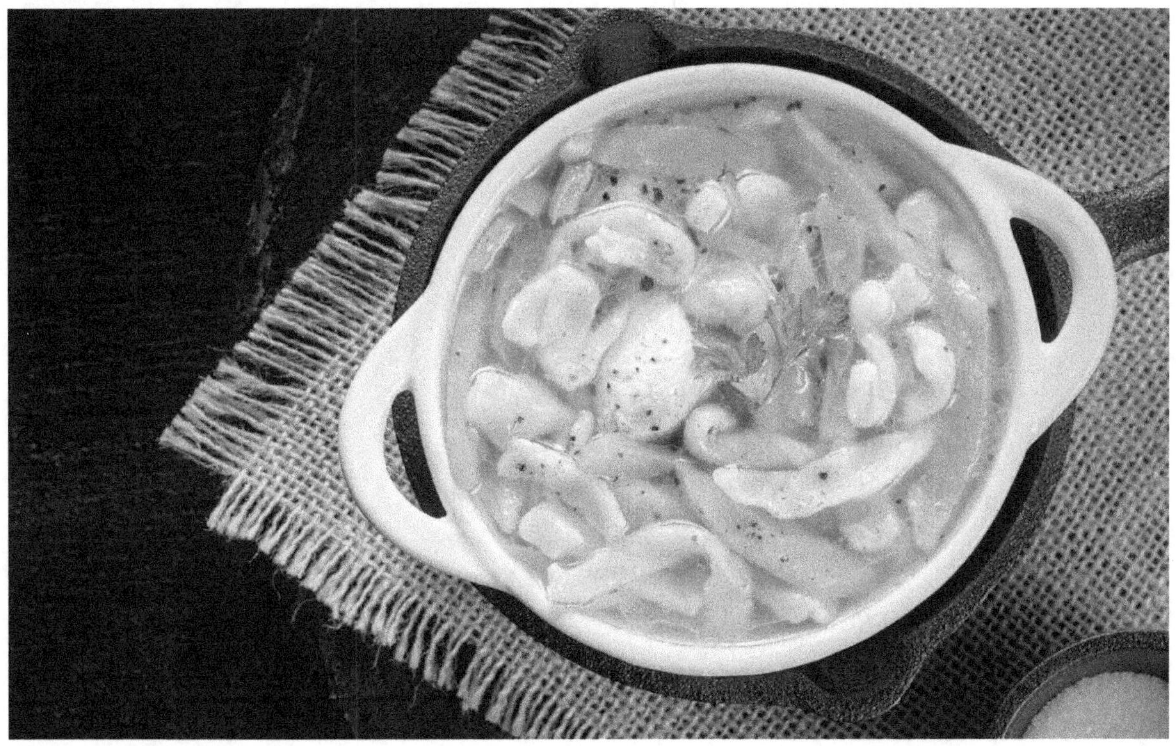

Here's a chicken soup dish infused with delightful Mediterranean flavors that you can't get enough of.

Serving Size: 6

Preparation & Cooking Time: 45 minutes

Ingredients:

- 2 tablespoons olive oil, divided
- ¾ lb. chicken breast fillets, sliced into cubes
- 1 onion, chopped
- 2 ribs celery, chopped
- 2 carrots, chopped
- ½ teaspoon dried oregano
- Salt and pepper to taste
- ¼ cup white wine
- 32 oz. low sodium chicken broth
- 1 teaspoon fresh rosemary, minced
- 1 bay leaf
- 1 cup orzo pasta (uncooked)
- 1 tablespoon lemon juice
- 1 teaspoon lemon zest
- Fresh parsley, minced

Instructions:

Pour 1 tablespoon olive oil into a pan over medium high heat.

Cook the chicken for 6 to 7 minutes.

Transfer the chicken to a plate.

Add the remaining olive oil to the pan.

Stir in the vegetables.

Season with the dried oregano, salt and pepper.

Cook while stirring for 5 minutes.

Pour in the wine and broth.

Add the rosemary and bay leaf.

Bring to a boil.

Next, add the orzo pasta.

Then, reduce heat and then simmer for 15 minutes or until the orzo is tender.

Add the chicken back to the pan.

Heat through for 5 minutes.

Stir in the lemon juice and lemon zest.

Discard the bay leaf.

Top with the parsley before serving.

16. Orange Salad with Poppy Seeds

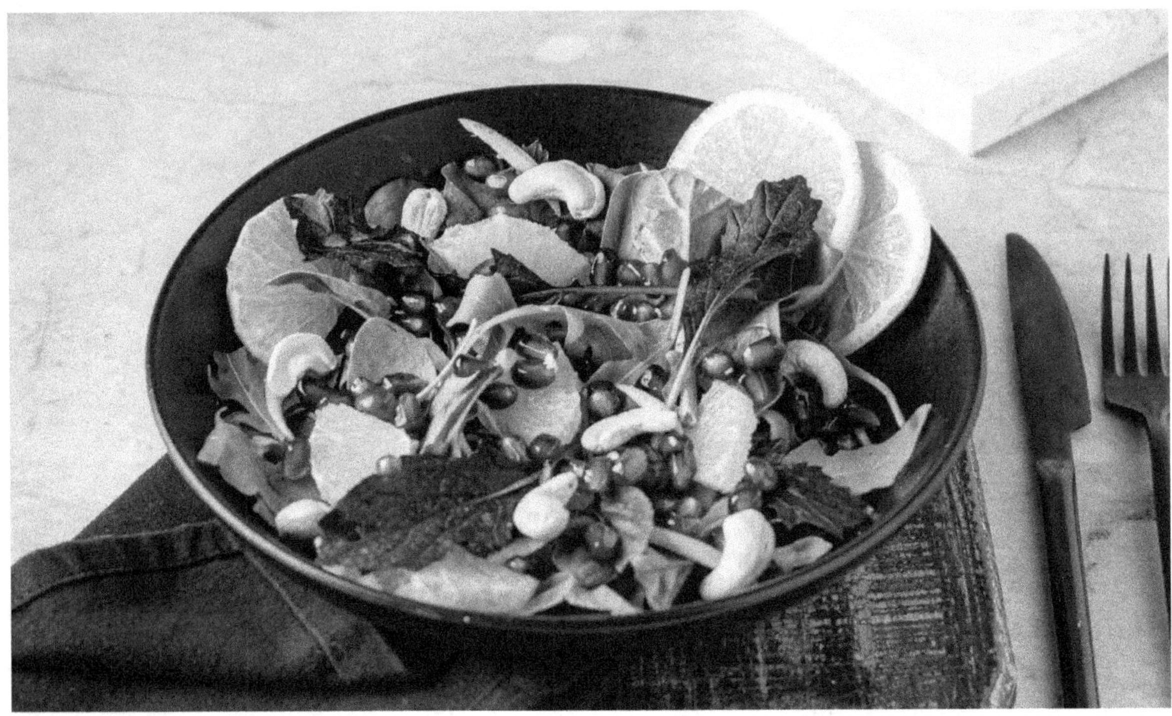

Here's a refreshing salad recipe that only takes a few minutes to prepare. You can prepare the salad dressing up to 3 days in advance. Just mix well before pouring over the salad.

Serving Size: 8

Preparation & Cooking Time: 40 minutes

Ingredients:

- 8 cups Romaine lettuce, shredded
- ¾ cup walnuts, chopped and toasted
- 15 oz. oranges, sliced
- 2/3 cup olive oil
- ¼ cup cider vinegar
- ½ cup sugar
- ½ teaspoon ground mustard
- 1 tablespoon poppy seeds
- ½ cup pomegranate seeds
- Salt to taste

Instructions:

Combine the Romaine lettuce, walnuts and oranges in a bowl.

In a small bowl, mix the olive oil, cider vinegar, sugar, ground mustard, poppy seeds, pomegranate seeds and salt.

Pour the mixture over the salad.

17. Chicken with Orange Salsa

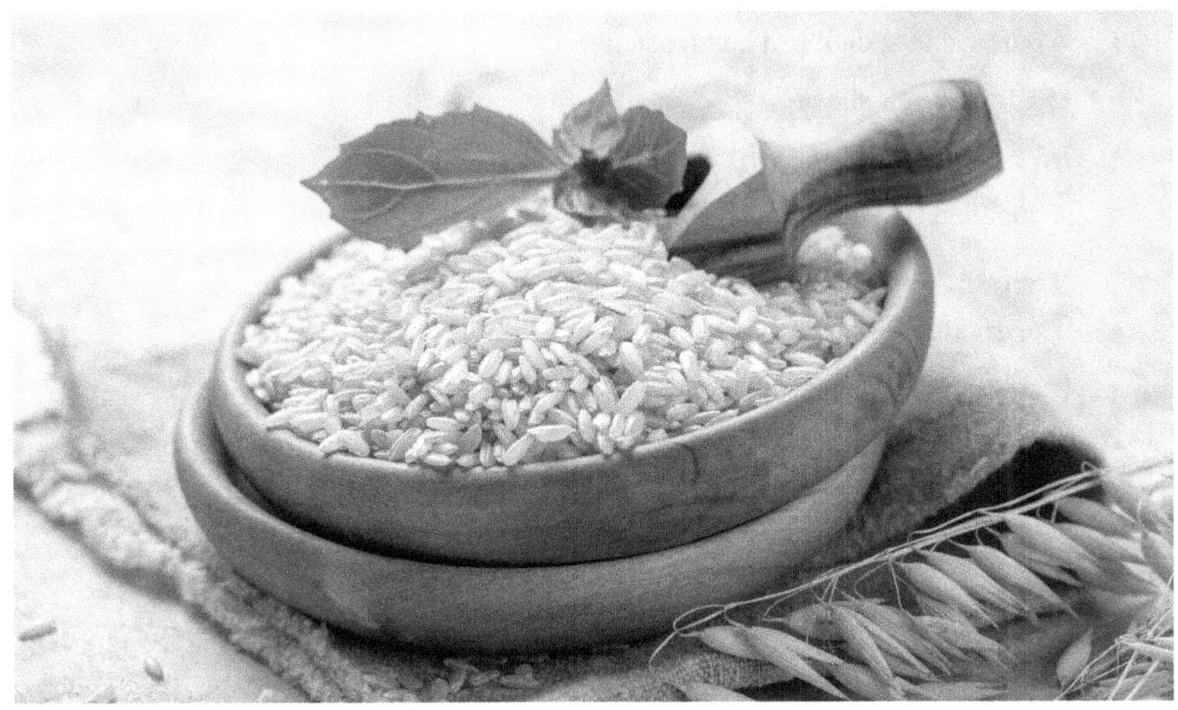

Flavor up chicken breast fillets with orange salsa! Even if you feel like you don't want to eat, this will surely bring back your appetite.

Serving Size: 4

Preparation & Cooking Time: 20 minutes

Ingredients:

- 1 tablespoon orange juice
- ¼ cup red onion, minced
- ½ cup pecans, chopped
- 2 tablespoons fresh cilantro, minced
- 1 lb. chicken breast fillets, sliced
- Salt and pepper to taste
- 1 tablespoon olive oil
- 2 cloves garlic, minced
- 4 cups cooked brown rice
- 11 oz. mandarin oranges, peeled and sliced

Instructions:

In a bowl, mix the orange juice, red onion, pecans and cilantro. Set aside.

Season the chicken with salt and pepper.

Pour the olive oil into a pan over medium high heat.

Cook the chicken for 4 minutes or until browned on both sides.

Add the garlic and orange juice mixture.

Bring to a boil.

Reduce heat and simmer for 5 minutes.

Serve the chicken with the salsa and rice, topped with the oranges.

18. Chicken & Turmeric Soup

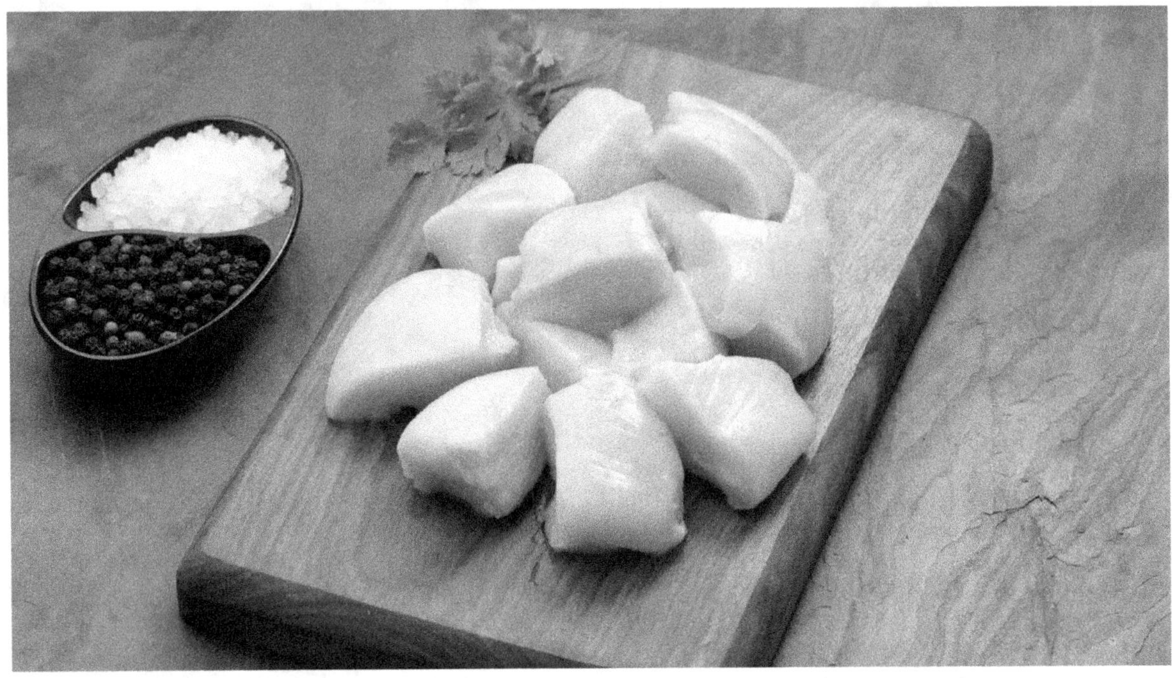

Turmeric is known for being anti-inflammatory as well as anti-infective. Adding turmeric powder to chicken soup can certainly enhance its nourishing and healing properties.

Serving Size: 4

Preparation & Cooking Time: 2 hours and 15 minutes

Ingredients:

- 16 cups water
- 1 head garlic, peeled and sliced horizontally
- 1 tablespoon ginger, sliced
- 3 lbs. chicken
- 1 tablespoon olive oil
- 1 red chili, minced
- 1 tablespoon garlic, minced
- 1 tablespoon ginger, minced
- 2 teaspoons turmeric powder
- 1 cup coconut milk
- ½ carrot, sliced into thin strips
- 1 tablespoon lime juice
- 1 tablespoon tamari
- Coriander sprigs

Instructions:

Pour the water into a pot over medium heat.

Add the garlic, ginger and chicken.

Bring to a boil.

Reduce heat and simmer for 1 hour and 30 minutes or until chicken is tender.

Skim the fat on the surface.

Transfer the chicken to a cutting board. Let cool.

Shred the chicken meat with a fork.

Discard the bones and skin.

Strain the chicken broth. Set aside.

Pour the coconut oil into a pan over medium heat.

Add the chili, garlic and ginger.

Cook while stirring for 2 minutes.

Add the turmeric.

Cook for another 1 minute.

Pour the chicken stock.

Add the chicken and carrot strips.

Stir in the lime juice and tamari.

Heat through for 5 minutes.

Ladle into soup bowls.

Top with the coriander sprigs.

19. Vegetarian Minestrone

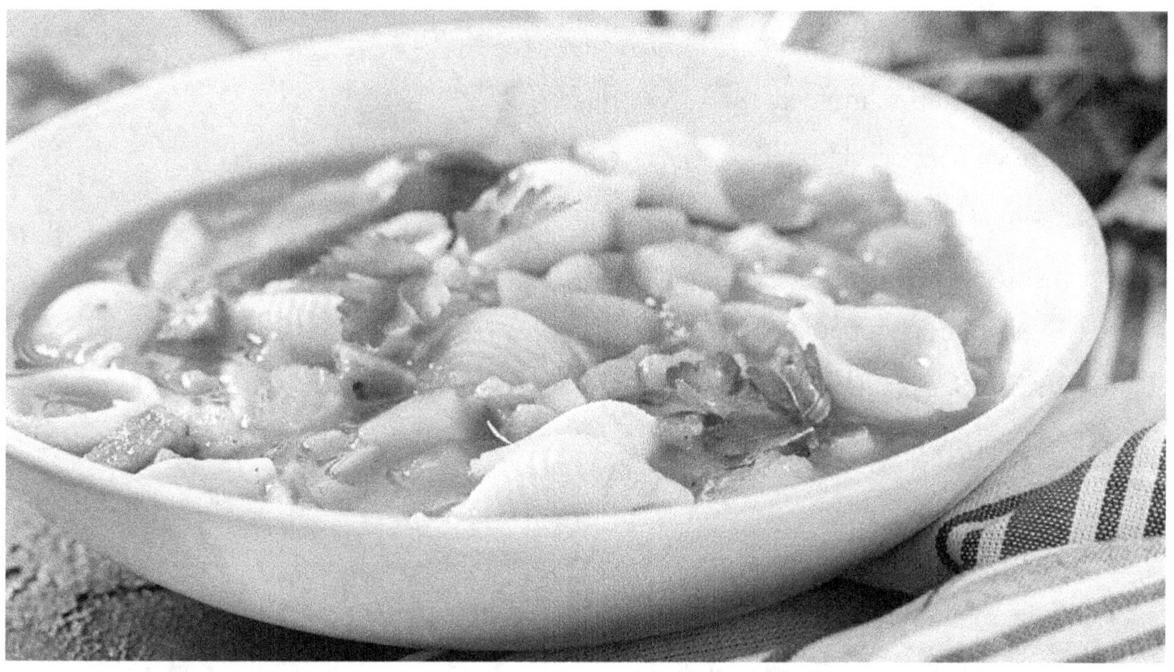

If you're looking for something light but tasty, here's a quick and easy minestrone recipe that you will surely enjoy.

Serving Size: 8

Preparation & Cooking Time: 1 hour and 10 minutes

Ingredients:

- 3 tablespoons olive oil
- 1 onion, chopped
- 6 cloves garlic, minced
- 1 green pepper, chopped
- 1 cup cabbage, chopped
- 2 carrots, chopped
- 1 zucchini, chopped
- 2 ribs celery, chopped
- 3 ½ cups water
- 15 oz. tomato puree
- 29 oz. canned diced tomatoes
- 8 oz. tomato sauce
- 15 oz. chickpeas, rinsed and drained
- 2 teaspoons dried basil
- 2 teaspoons dried oregano
- 3 tablespoons dried parsley flakes
- ¼ teaspoon cayenne pepper
- Salt and pepper to taste
- ½ cup pasta shells

For serving

- Fresh basil leaves
- Parmesan cheese, shaved

Instructions:

Add the olive oil to a pan over medium heat.

Cook the onion, garlic, green pepper, cabbage, carrots, zucchini and celery for 3 minutes.

Pour in the water, tomato puree, canned diced tomatoes and tomato sauce.

Add the chickpeas.

Season with the dried herbs, cayenne pepper, salt and pepper.

Bring to a boil.

Reduce heat and simmer for 15 minutes.

Add the pasta.

Cook for 15 minutes.

Ladle into soup bowls.

Garnish with the basil and Parmesan cheese.

20. Mixed Green Salad with Orange Vinaigrette

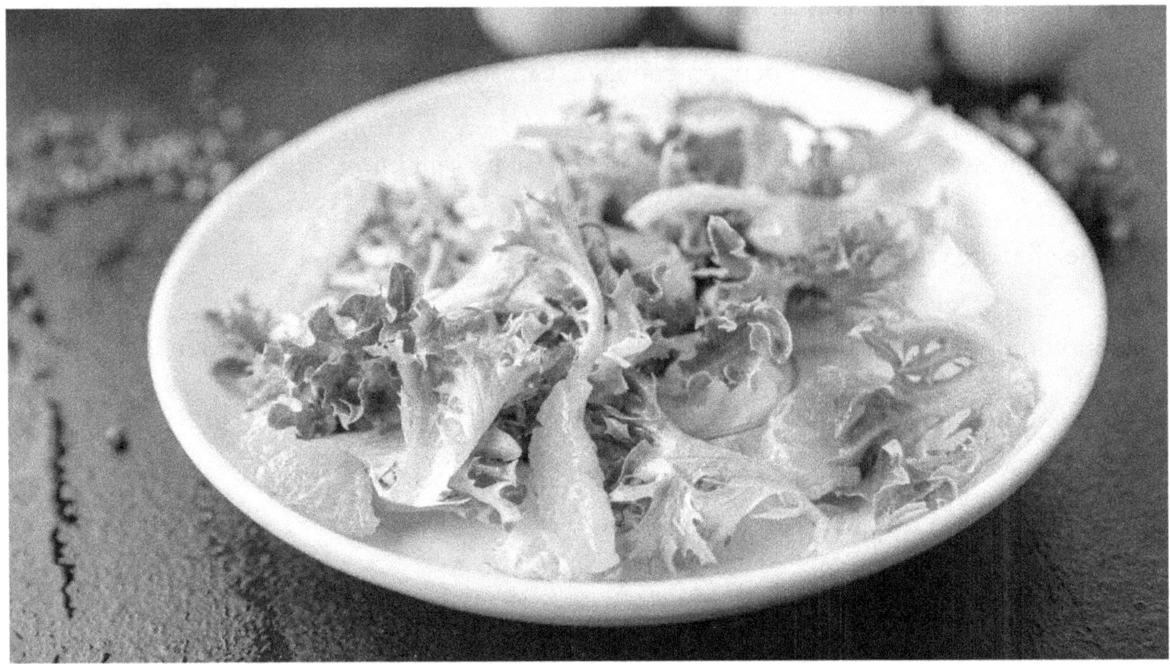

Whisk together mixed salad greens, oranges, onions and apples, drizzle with dressing, and that's it! You have a light and healthy lunch you can enjoy after just a few minutes.

Serving Size: 8

Preparation & Cooking Time: 20 minutes

Ingredients:

Dressing

- ¼ cup canola oil
- 2 tablespoons white vinegar
- ¼ cup orange juice
- 2 teaspoons ginger, grated
- 2 tablespoons honey
- ¼ teaspoon cayenne pepper
- Salt to taste

Salad

- 12 cups mixed salad greens
- 2 oranges, peeled and sliced
- 1 cup red onion, sliced thinly

Instructions:

Combine the canola oil, white vinegar, orange juice, ginger, honey, cayenne pepper and salt in a glass jar.

Seal the jar and shake.

In a serving bowl, toss together the salad greens, oranges and red onion.

Drizzle with the dressing and serve.

21. Pumpkin Bisque

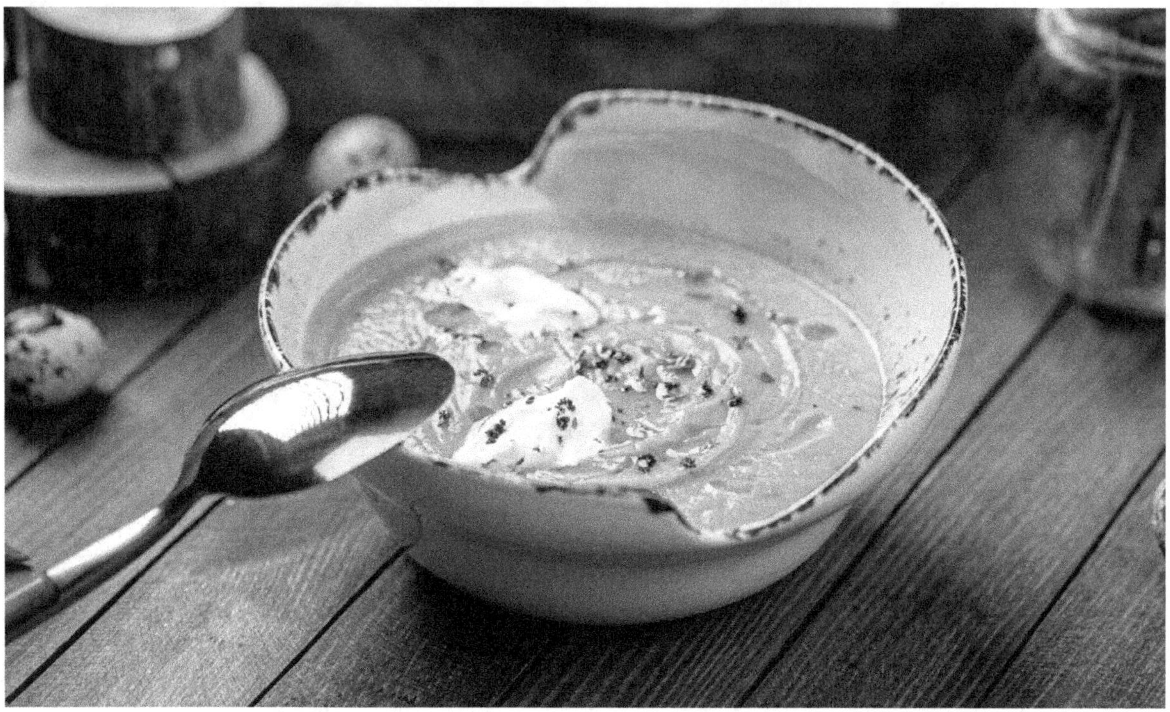

Here's a pumpkin bisque recipe made extra special with gouda cheese. You will definitely savor each sip.

Serving Size: 8

Preparation & Cooking Time: 1 hour

Ingredients:

- 4 strips bacon, chopped
- 1 onion, chopped
- 3 cloves garlic, minced
- 6 cups chicken broth
- 29 oz. pumpkin puree
- ¼ teaspoon ground nutmeg
- Salt and pepper to taste
- 1 cup heavy whipping cream
- 1 cup gouda cheese, shredded
- 2 tablespoons fresh parsley, minced

Instructions:

Add the bacon to a pan over medium heat.

Cook until crispy.

Drain the bacon in a plate lined with paper towels.

Transfer to a cutting board and mince.

Cook the onion in the bacon drippings until tender.

Next, add the garlic and cook for another 1 minute.

Pour in the chicken broth.

Add the pumpkin puree.

Season with the ground nutmeg, salt and pepper.

Bring to a boil.

Reduce heat and simmer for 10 minutes.

Let cool for 5 minutes.

Process the mixture in a blender until smooth.

Add the mixture to a pot.

Stir in the cream.

Heat through for 5 minutes.

Add the gouda cheese and cook while stirring until melted.

Top the soup with the bacon and parsley.

22. Carrot Chowder

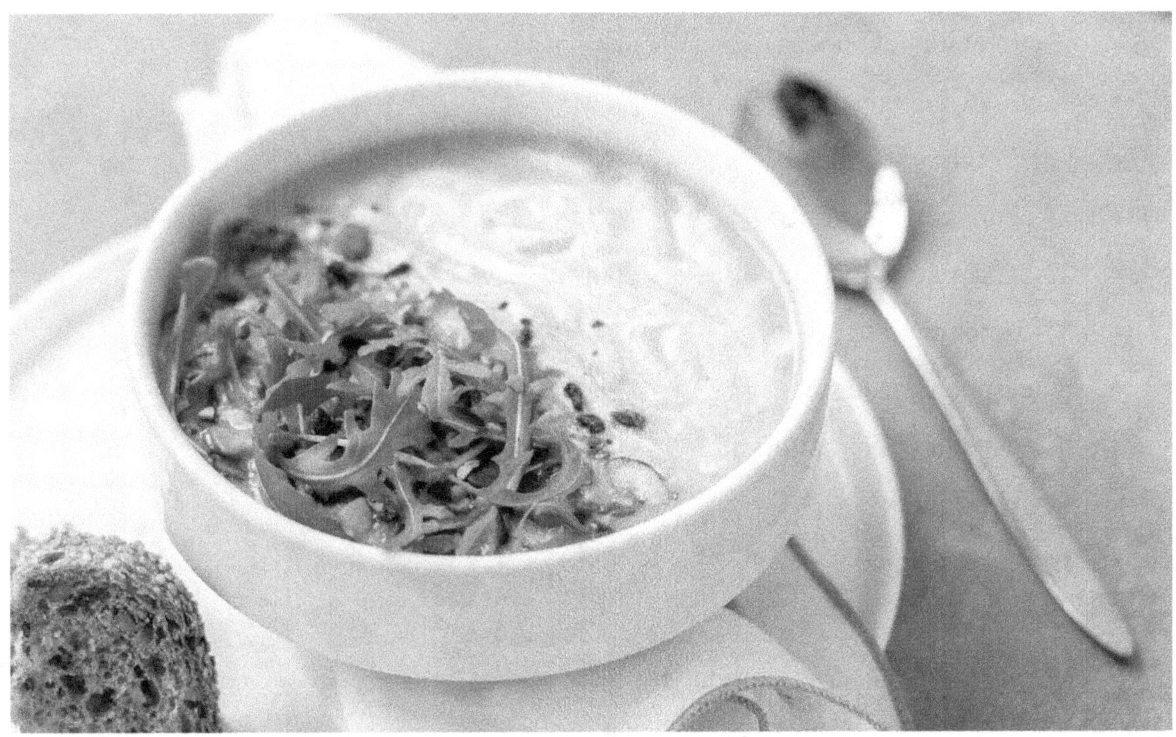

This buttermilk pie crust is an alternative to the traditional pastry crust. Additional ingredients like buttermilk and butter give this pie crust a delicious buttery flavor. To make this recipe extra

Serving Size: 10

Preparation & Cooking Time: 1 hour and 20 minutes

Ingredients:

- 1 lb. ground beef, cooked and drained
- ½ cup onion, chopped
- 1 cup green pepper, chopped
- ½ cup celery, chopped
- 2 ½ cups carrots, grated
- 22 oz. condensed cream of celery soup
- 32 oz. tomato juice
- ½ teaspoon garlic salt
- ½ teaspoon dried marjoram
- 1 ½ cups water
- 1 teaspoon sugar
- Salt to taste
- Monterey Jack cheese, shredded

Instructions:

Add all the ingredients except the Monterey Jack cheese to a pot over medium heat.

Bring to a boil.

Reduce heat and simmer for 1 hour.

Ladle into soup bowls.

Top with the shredded cheese before serving.

23. Tomato Soup

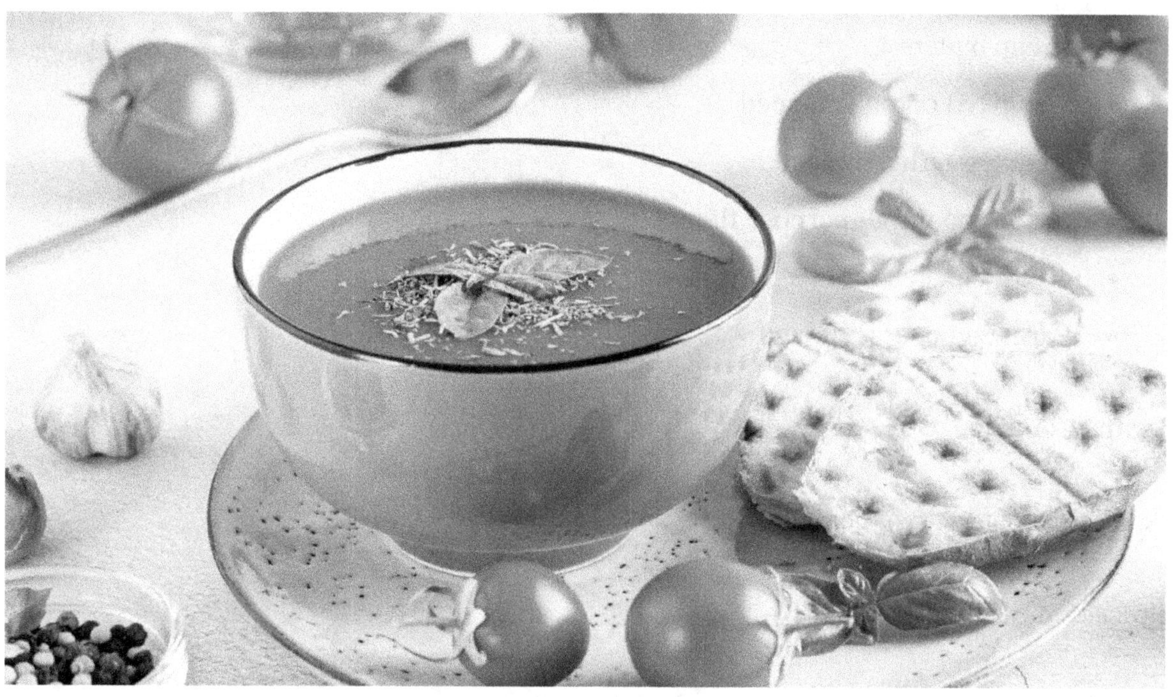

Here's another comfort food that you'd be craving for when you're not feeling so well. This will immediately give you relief.

Serving Size: 8

Preparation & Cooking Time: 30 minutes

Ingredients:

- 14 oz. canned diced tomatoes with herbs and garlic
- ¼ cup butter
- ½ cup red onion, chopped
- 2 cloves garlic, minced
- 6 tablespoons all purpose flour
- 48 oz. chicken broth
- Parmesan cheese, grated

Instructions:

Add the tomatoes to a blender.

Process until smooth.

Add the butter to a pan over medium high heat.

Cook the onion and garlic until tender.

Add the flour.

Cook while stirring for 1 hour.

Pour in the tomatoes and chicken broth.

Bring to a boil.

Reduce heat and simmer for 20 minutes.

Top with the cheese before serving.

24. Ambrosia Salad

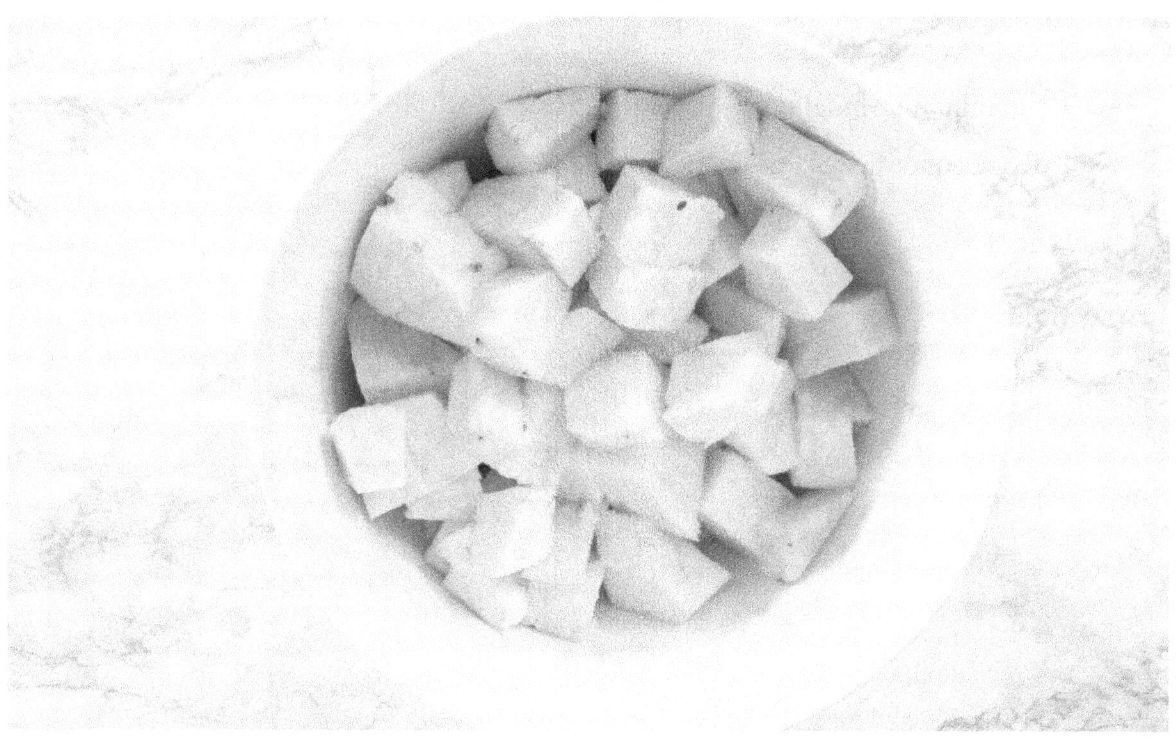

This fruit medley is a great idea whether you're having the sniffles or you just want a quick and healthy snack to cheer you up. You'll only need 5 ingredients to prepare this creamy and refreshing salad.

Serving Size: 4

Preparation & Cooking Time: 2 hours and 10 minutes

Ingredients:

- 15 oz. oranges, peeled and sliced
- 8 oz. pineapple chunks
- 1 cup mini marshmallows
- 1 cup coconut flakes (sweetened)
- 1 cup sour cream

Instructions:

Mix all the ingredients in a bowl.

Cover and refrigerate for 2 hours.

Serve.

25. Vegetable Soup

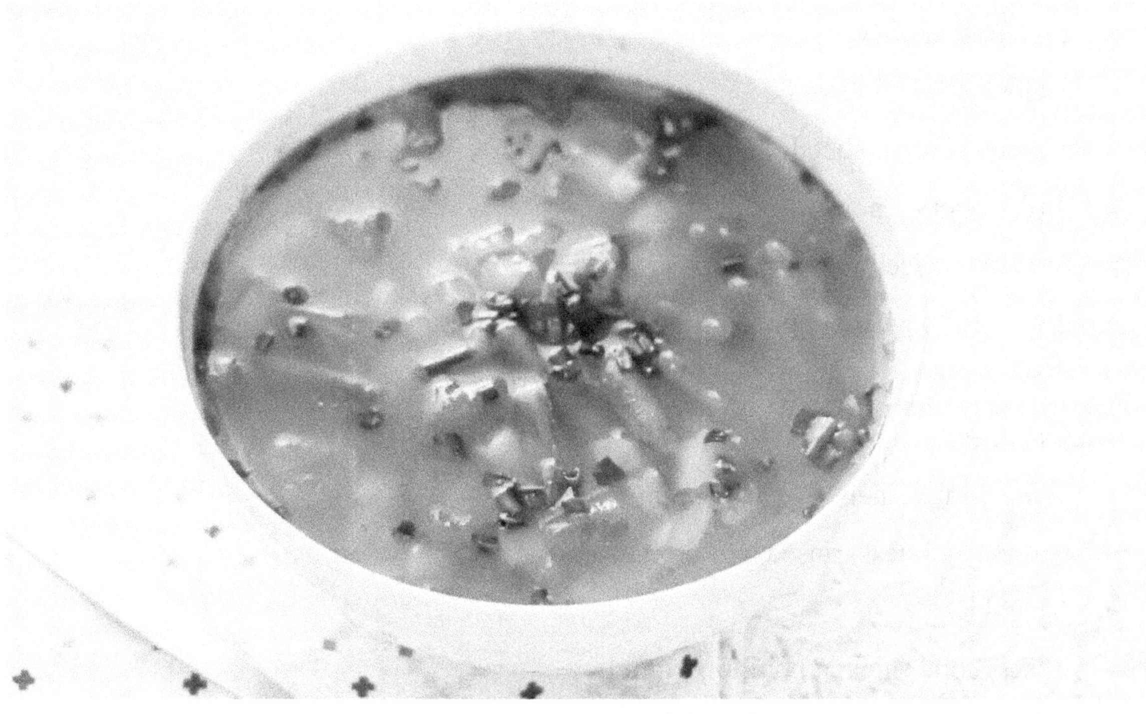

This is an immune-boosting vegetable soup recipe that you can make when you feel like you're about to go down with a flu.

Serving Size: 16

Preparation & Cooking Time: 1 hour and 45 minutes

Ingredients:

- 1 tablespoon olive oil
- 2 onions, chopped
- 1 clove garlic, minced
- 1 green pepper, sliced
- 4 ribs celery, chopped
- 8 carrots, sliced
- 2 cups cabbage, chopped
- 8 oz. green beans
- 8 oz. peas
- 1 cup corn kernels
- 15 oz. chickpeas, rinsed and drained
- 1 bay leaf
- 2 teaspoons chicken bouillon granules
- 1 ½ teaspoons dried parsley flakes
- 1 teaspoon dried marjoram
- 1 teaspoon dried thyme
- ½ teaspoon dried basil
- Salt and pepper to taste
- 4 cups water
- 28 oz. canned diced tomatoes
- 2 cups vegetable juice

Instructions:

Add the olive oil to a pot over medium heat.

Cook the onion, garlic, green pepper, celery and carrots until tender.

Stir in the garlic.

Cook for 1 minute.

Add the remaining ingredients.

Bring to a boil.

Reduce heat and simmer for 1 hour and 30 minutes.

Discard the bay leaf before serving.

26. Fruit Cup

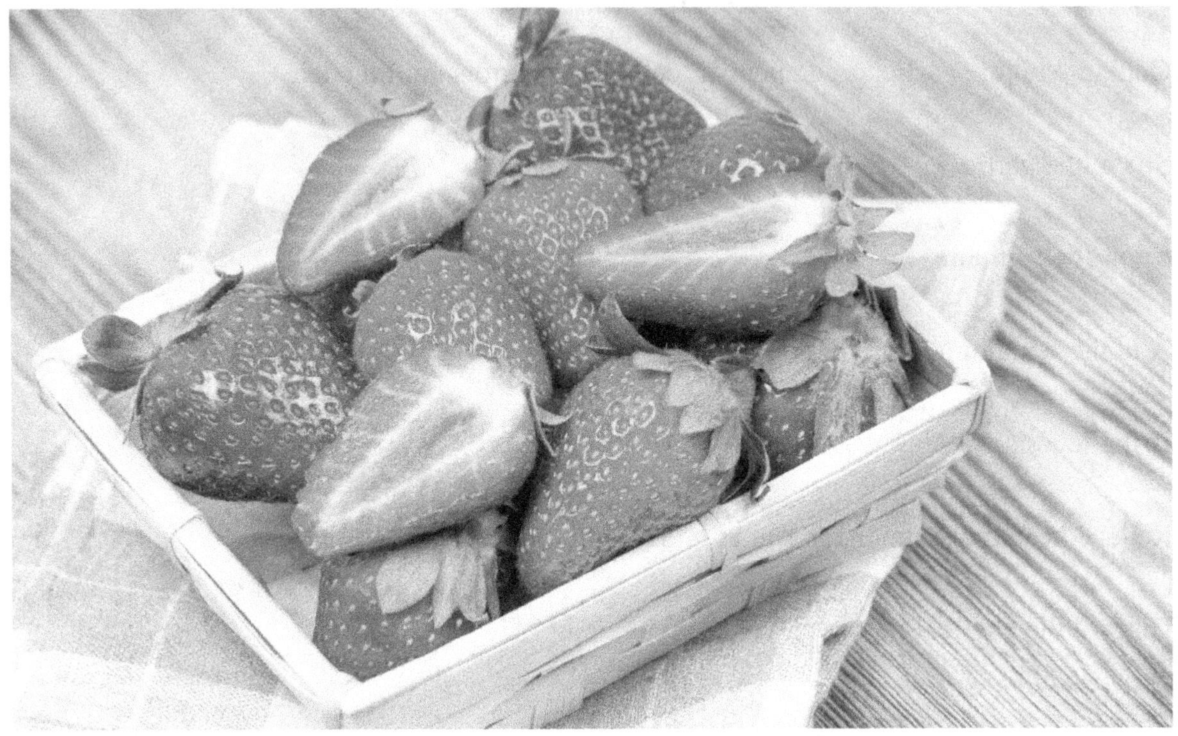

You'll love this vibrant and flavorful fruit cup which is also a cinch to prepare.

Serving Size: 6

Preparation & Cooking Time: 2 hours and 10 minutes

Ingredients:

- 2 tablespoons lemon juice
- ¼ cup grape juice
- ¾ cup orange juice
- 1 tablespoon sugar
- 1 cup fresh strawberries, sliced in half
- 1 cup green grapes, sliced in half
- 1 ½ cups cantaloupe balls

Garnish

- Fresh mint leaves

Instructions:

In a bowl, mix the lemon juice, grape juice, orange juice and sugar.

In a serving bowl, combine the strawberries, grapes and cantaloupe balls.

Pour the juice mixture into the bowl with fruits.

Toss to combine.

Cover the bowl.

Refrigerate for 2 hours.

Top with the mint leaves before serving.

27. Ginger & Kale Smoothie

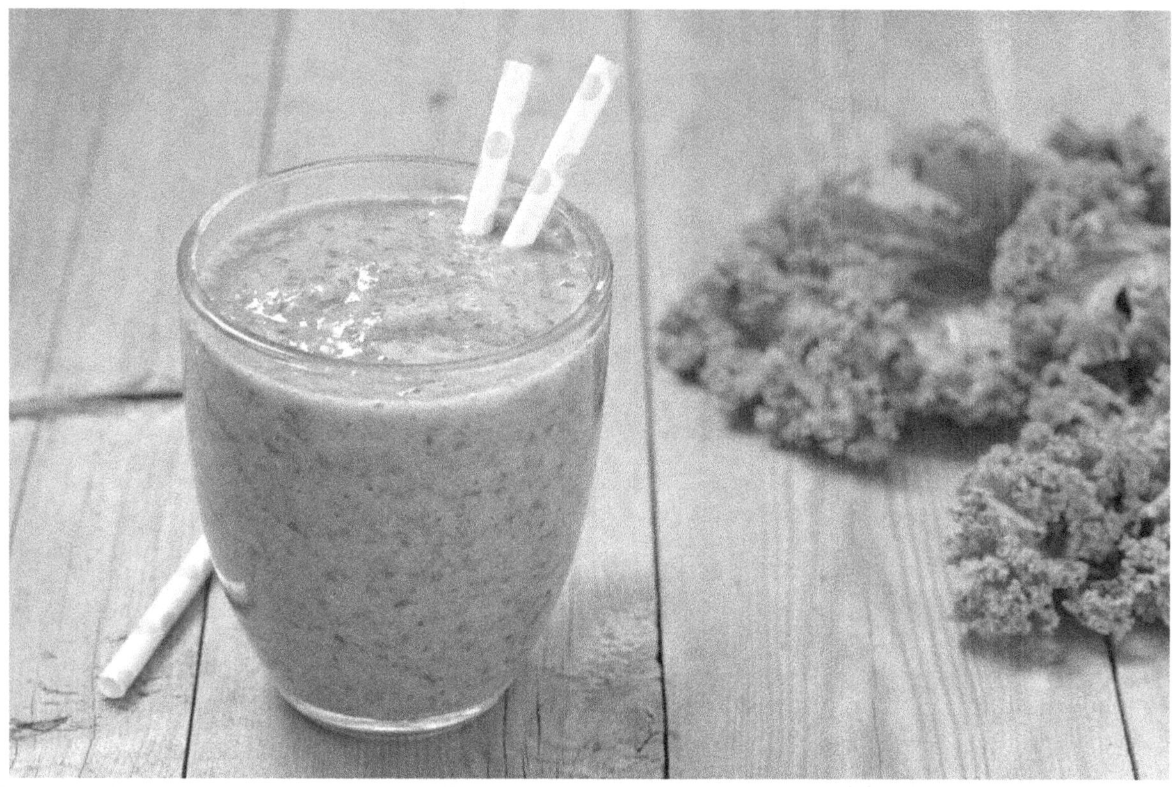

Ginger and kale are both known for their anti-viral, antibacterial and immune-boosting properties. So if you feel like you're coming down with a cold or flu, take out the blender and make yourself this delicious smoothie.

Serving Size: 2

Preparation & Cooking Time: 15 minutes

Ingredients:

- 1 ¼ cups orange juice
- 1 teaspoon lemon juice
- 2 cups fresh kale leaves
- 1 apple, peeled and chopped
- 1 tablespoon ginger, minced
- 4 ice cubes
- 1/8 teaspoon ground cinnamon
- 1/8 teaspoon ground turmeric
- Pinch cayenne pepper

Instructions:

Add all the ingredients in a blender.

Cover.

Process until blended.

Pour the mixture into glasses and serve.

28. Chicken Stir Fry with Honey

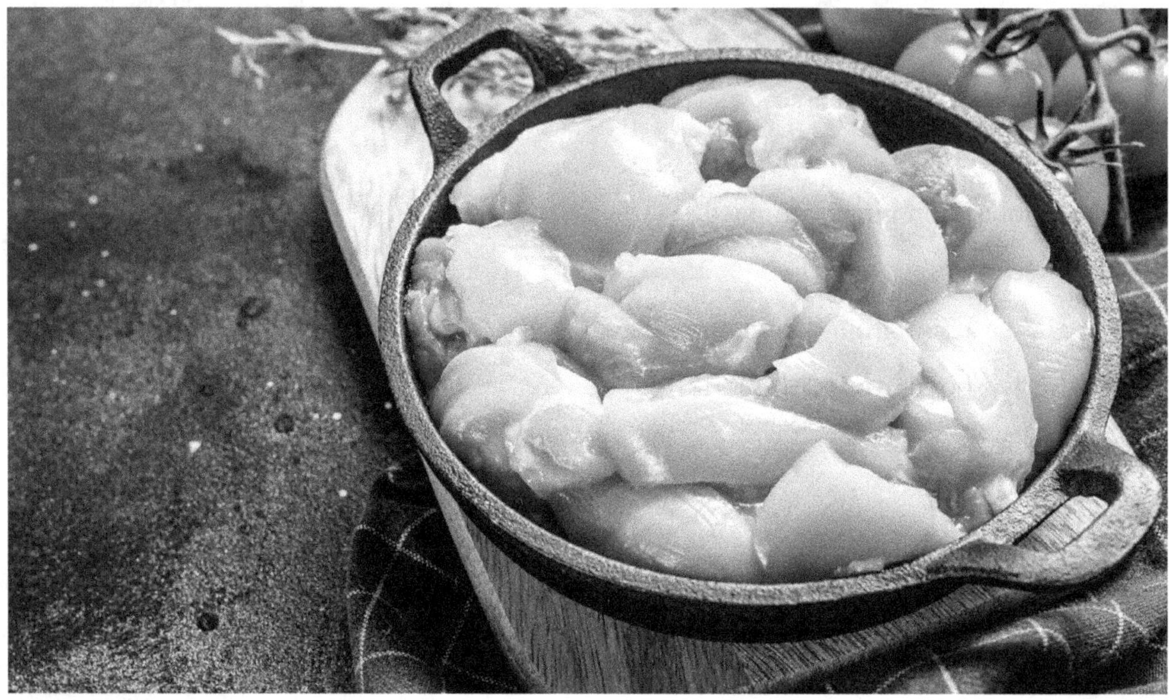

If you like meals that are ready in no time, here's a chicken stir fry dish that you can make. It's made with few ingredients, and takes minimal effort to prepare.

Serving Size: 4

Preparation & Cooking Time: 30 minutes

Ingredients:

- 3 teaspoons olive oil, divided
- 1 clove garlic, minced
- 1 lb. chicken breast fillets, sliced into cubes
- 2 tablespoons low sodium soy sauce
- 3 tablespoons honey
- Salt and pepper to taste
- 16 oz. frozen stir-fry vegetable mix
- 2 teaspoons cornstarch
- 1 tablespoon cold water

Instructions:

Add 2 tablespoons olive oil to a pan over medium high heat.

Cook the garlic and chicken for 1 minute, stirring often.

In a bowl, mix the soy sauce, honey, salt and pepper.

Cook while stirring for 2 minutes.

Transfer to a plate.

Pour the remaining olive oil into the pan.

Add the vegetable mix.

In a small bowl, mix the cornstarch and water.

Add the cornstarch mixture and chicken to the pan.

Bring to a boil.

Cook until the sauce has thickened.

29. Gingered Brussels Sprouts

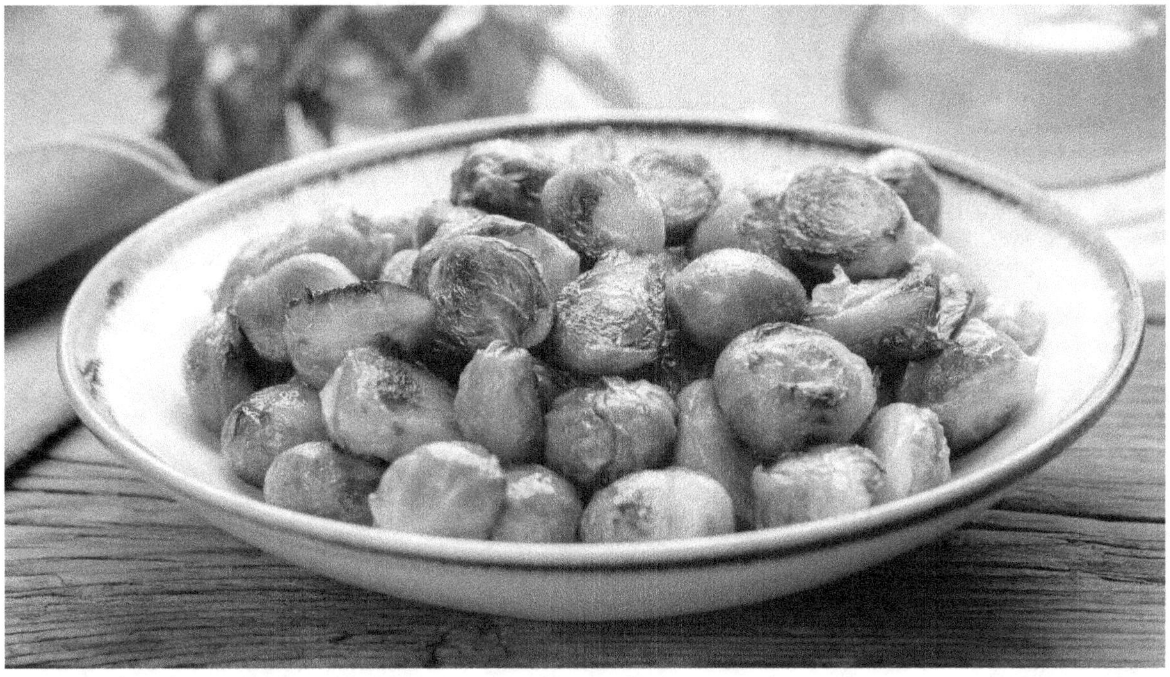

You're going to enjoy this dish that you can make without too much fuss.

Serving Size: 6

Preparation & Cooking Time: 30 minutes

Ingredients:

- 1 tablespoon olive oil
- 1 onion, minced
- 1 clove garlic, minced
- 1 tablespoon ginger, minced
- 1 lb. Brussels sprouts, trimmed and sliced thinly
- 2 tablespoons water
- Salt and pepper to taste

Instructions:

Add the oil to a pan over medium heat.

Cook the onion, garlic and ginger for 2 to 3 minutes, stirring often.

Stir in the Brussels sprouts.

Cook until tender.

Pour in the water.

Simmer for 1 minute.

Season with salt and pepper.

30. Turkey Minestrone

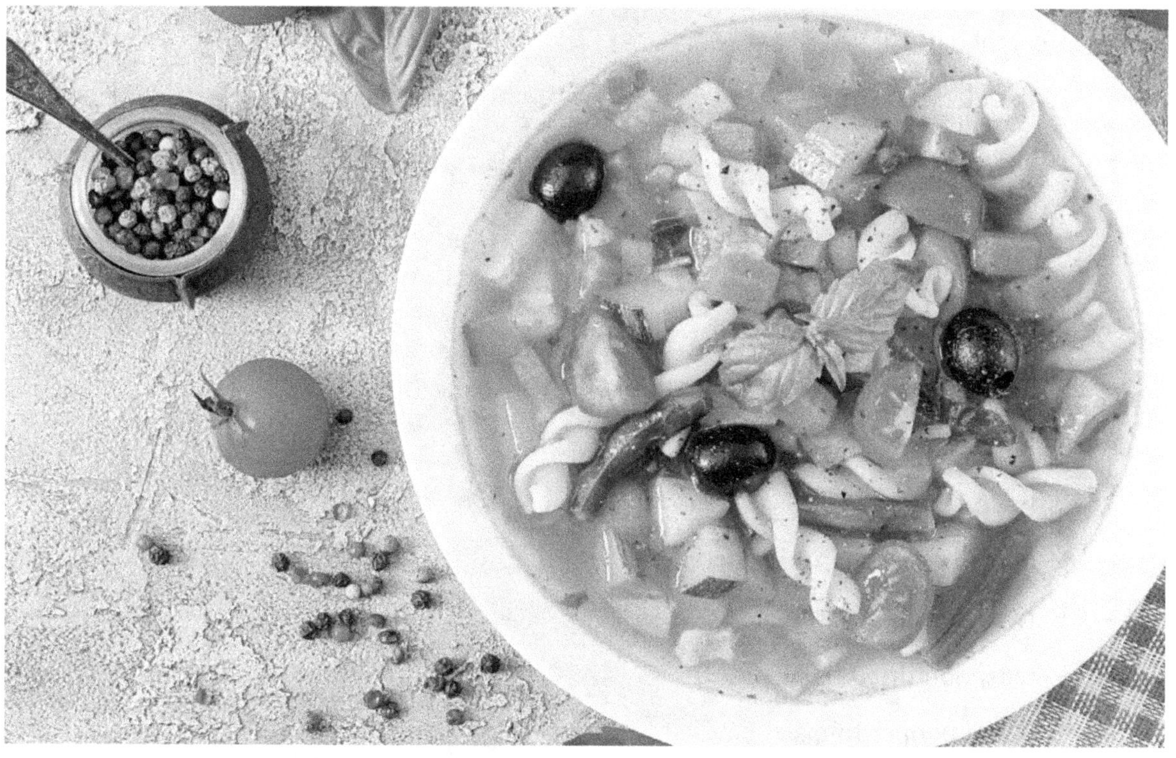

Here's a great idea if you have leftover turkey at home that you don't know what to do with. And if you or anyone in the family is not feeling well, this dish can surely help.

Serving Size: 6

Preparation & Cooking Time: 30 minutes

Ingredients:

- 1 tablespoon olive oil
- 1 carrot, sliced
- 1 rib celery, sliced
- 1 clove garlic, minced
- 14 ½ oz. canned diced tomatoes
- 4 cups chicken broth
- 2/3 cup corn
- 2/3 cup green peas
- 1 onion, chopped
- 2/3 cup green beans
- ½ cup elbow macaroni (uncooked)
- ¼ teaspoon dried oregano
- ¼ teaspoon dried basil
- Salt and pepper to taste
- 1 bay leaf
- 1 cup turkey, cooked and sliced into cubes
- 1 zucchini, peeled and sliced
- ¼ cup Parmesan cheese, grated

Instructions:

Pour the olive oil into a pan over medium high heat.

Cook the onion, garlic, celery and carrot until tender.

Pour in the canned diced tomatoes and chicken broth.

Stir in the corn, green peas and green beans.

Add the macaroni, dried oregano, dried basil, salt and pepper.

Bring to a boil.

Reduce heat and simmer for 5 minutes

Stir in the turkey.

Add the zucchini.

Discard bay leaf.

Cook until the zucchini is tender but still crispy.

Top with the cheese before serving.

31. Chicken & Vegetable Pasta

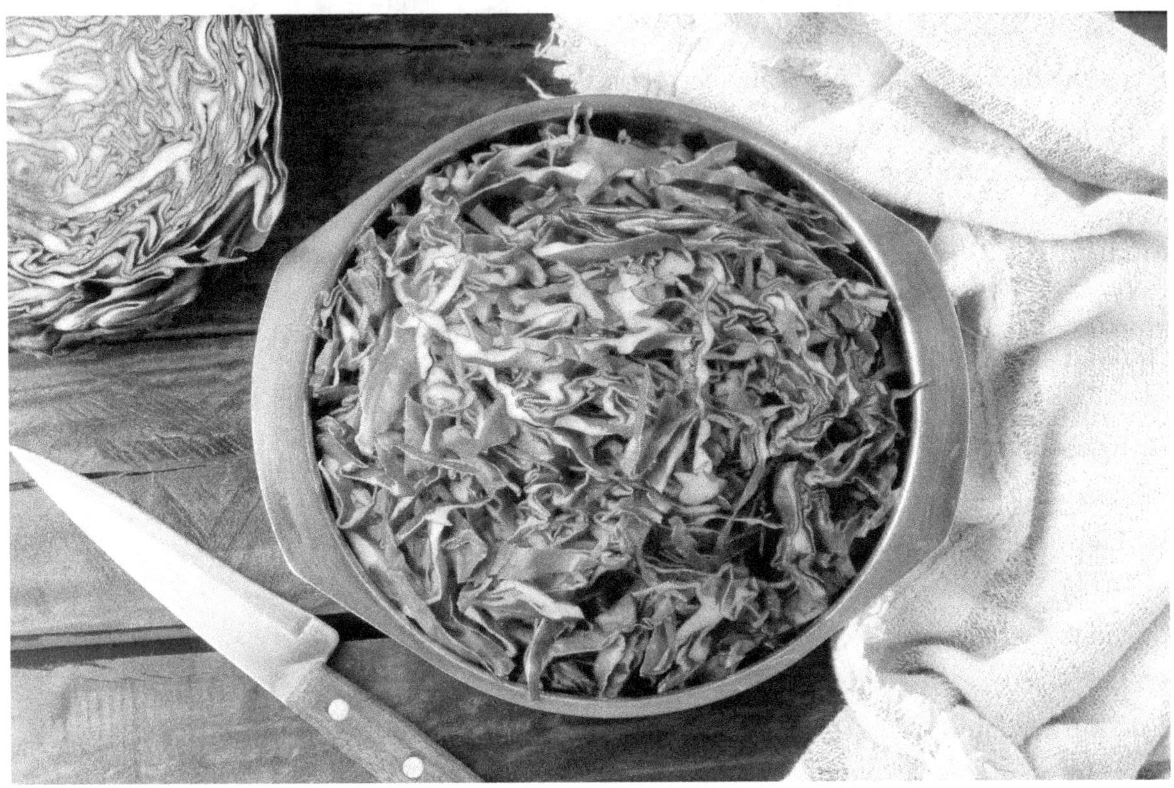

Toss pasta in a handful of bright vegetables and cooked chicken for a quick and easy lunch idea.

Serving Size: 8

Preparation & Cooking Time: 30 minutes

Ingredients:

- 2 cups elbow pasta
- 1 tablespoon coconut oil
- ½ red onion, sliced
- 2 teaspoons garlic paste
- 2 teaspoons ginger paste
- ½ sweet red pepper, chopped
- ½ cup red cabbage, chopped
- 1 ½ cups Brussels sprouts, chopped
- ½ cup carrots, shredded
- Pinch chili pepper
- Salt and pepper to taste
- 1 rotisserie chicken, shredded
- 2 green onions, minced

Instructions:

Prepare the pasta according to the directions in the package.

Rinse, drain and set aside.

Pour the coconut oil into a pan over medium heat.

Cook the onion, garlic paste and ginger paste for 1 to 2 minutes.

Stir in the sweet red pepper, red cabbage, Brussels sprouts and carrots.

Season with the chili pepper, salt and pepper.

Cook for 5 to 7 minutes or until vegetables are tender but still crispy.

Add the chicken.

Heat through for 3 minutes.

Toss the pasta into the mixture.

Turn off heat.

Transfer pasta into a serving bowl or platter.

Sprinkle the green onions on top and serve.

32. Berry & Yogurt Pops

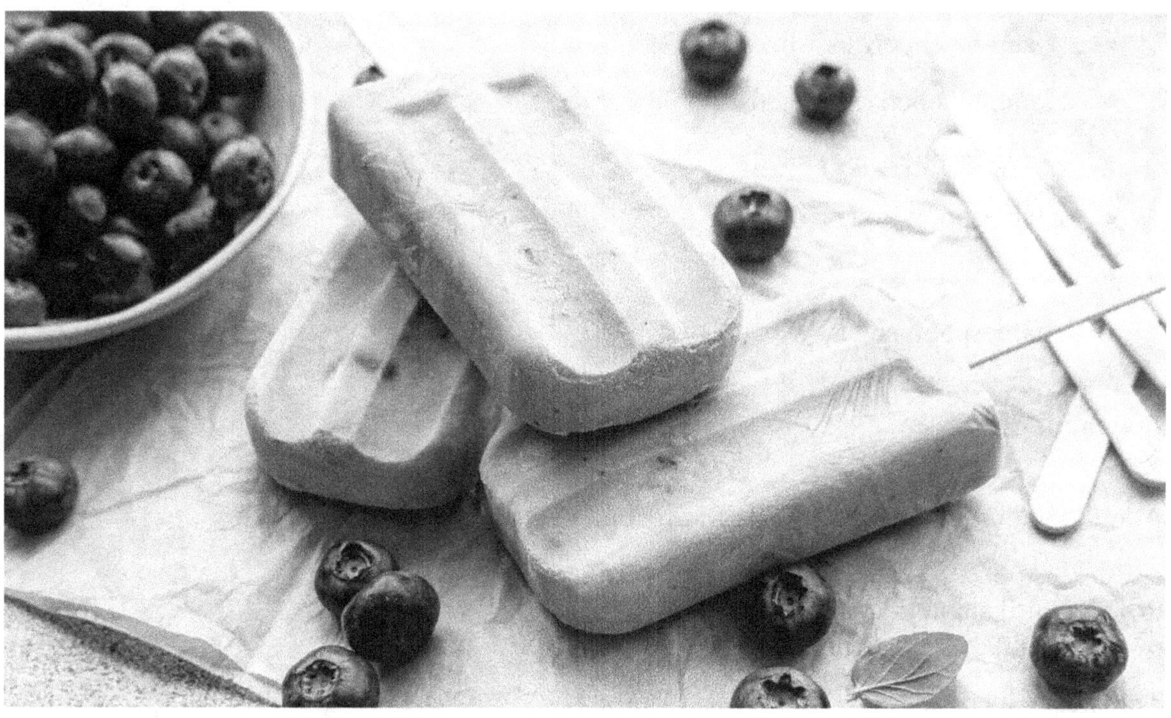

Here's a refreshing snack idea that would take your mind off your cold or flu—berry and yogurt pops!

Serving Size: 4

Preparation & Cooking Time: 2 hours and 10 minutes

Ingredients:

- 2 ¾ cups nonfat Greek yogurt
- ¼ cup blackberries, sliced
- ¼ cup blueberries, sliced
- ¼ cup raspberries, sliced
- 1 tablespoon honey
- ¼ cup water
- 1 tablespoon sugar

Instructions:

Add the yogurt and berries to a food processor or blender.

Process until smooth.

Transfer to a bowl.

Stir in the honey, water and sugar.

Transfer to popsicle molds.

Freeze for 2 hours or until firm.

33. Carrot Casserole

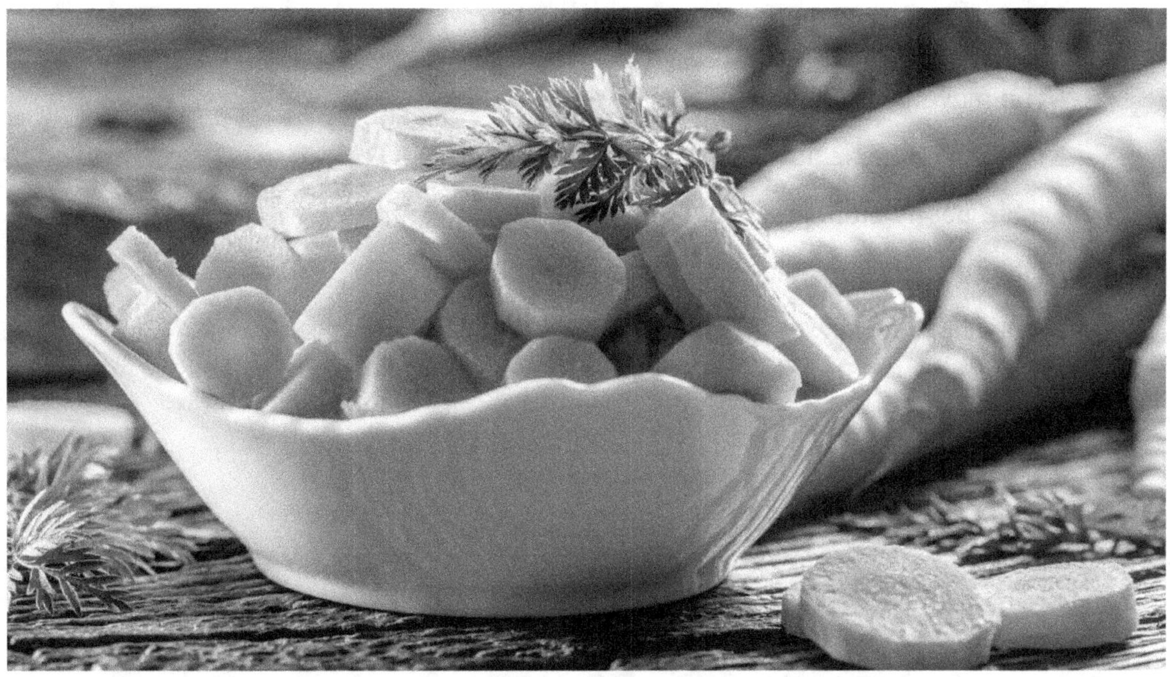

This dish is so delicious even those who don't like carrots will probably be back for another serving. This is also a great idea if you're coming down with a cold or flu as carrots are packed with vitamins and antioxidants that can boost your body's immune resistance.

Serving Size: 8

Preparation & Cooking Time: 45 minutes

Ingredients:

- 1 cup water
- 1 ½ lb. carrots, sliced
- 1 cup mayonnaise
- 1 tablespoon horseradish
- 1 tablespoon onion, grated
- 2 tablespoons plain crackers, crushed
- ¼ cup cheddar cheese, shredded

Instructions:

Preheat your oven to 350 degrees F.

Pour the water into a pan over medium heat.

Add the carrots.

Bring to a boil.

Reduce heat and simmer for 8 minutes.

Drain the carrots but reserve ¼ cup of the cooking liquid.

Transfer to a baking pan.

In a bowl, mix the cooking liquid, mayo, horseradish and onion.

Spread the mixture on top of the carrots.

Top with the crackers and cheese.

Bake in the oven for 30 minutes.

34. Green Beans with Garlic & Bacon

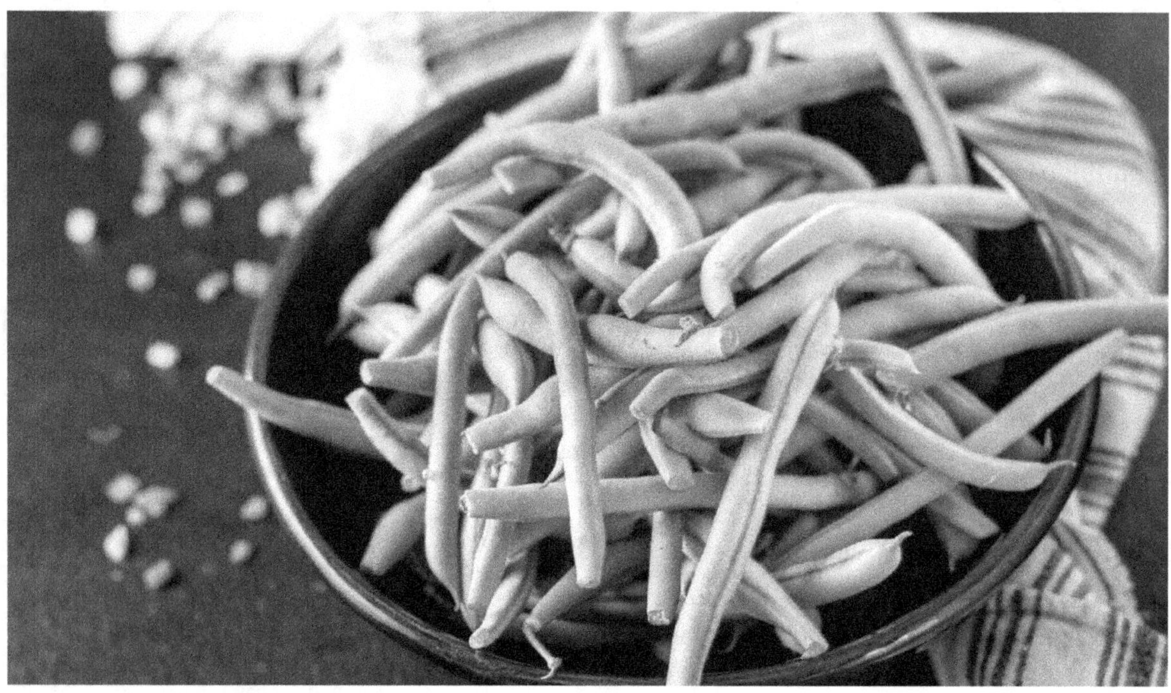

Bacon can help cheer you up even when you're feeling ill. But be sure to combine bacon with something healthy and nutritious like garlic and green beans!

Serving Size: 8

Preparation & Cooking Time: 30 minutes

Ingredients:

- 6 strips bacon strips, chopped
- 1 tablespoon olive oil
- 6 tablespoons butter
- 1 onion, sliced thinly
- 3 cloves garlic, minced
- ¼ cup chicken broth
- 9 cups green beans, trimmed and sliced
- ½ teaspoon garlic powder
- Salt and pepper to taste
- 2 tablespoons lemon juice

Instructions:

Add the bacon to a pan over medium heat.

Cook until crispy.

Transfer the bacon strips to a plate lined with paper towels.

Add the olive oil and butter to the same pan.

Cook the onion and garlic for 1 to 2 minutes, stirring often.

Pour in the chicken broth.

Bring to a boil.

Simmer for 5 minutes or until cooking liquid is reduced to half.

Add the green beans.

Season with the garlic powder, salt and pepper.

Heat through for 3 to 5 minutes.

Drizzle with the lemon juice before serving.

35. Garlic Roasted Vegetables

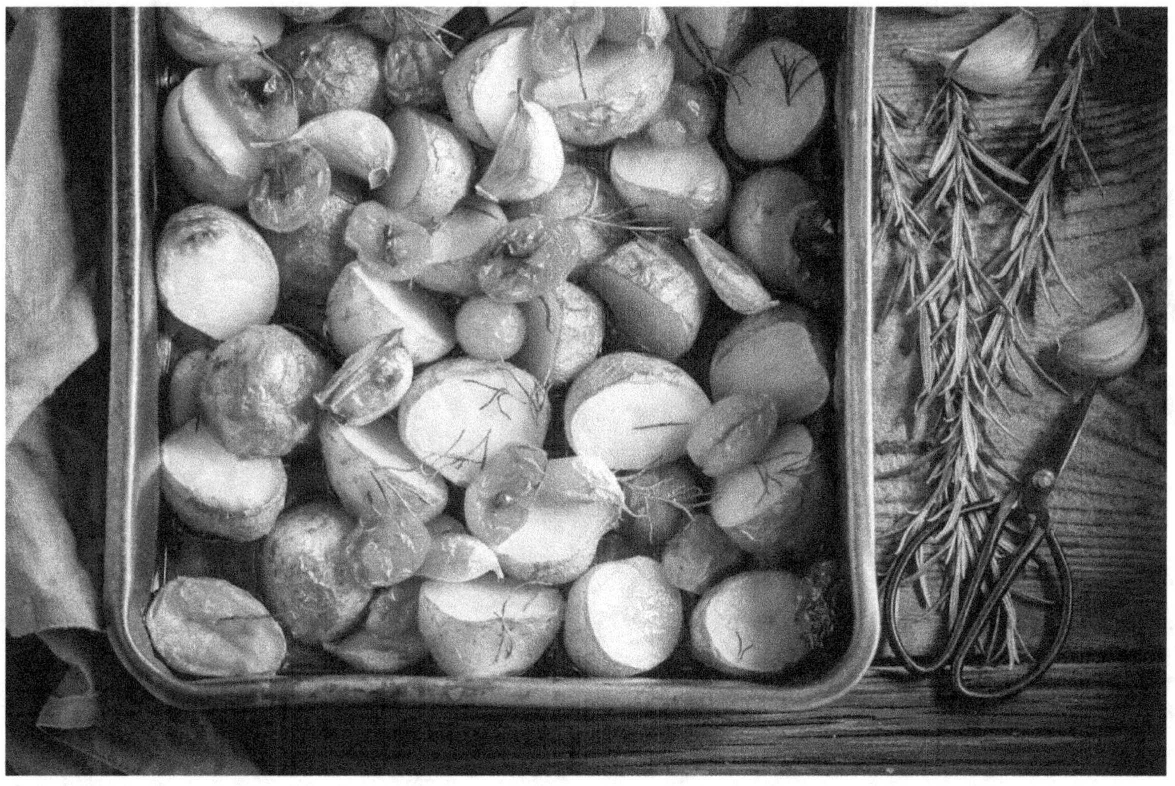

Herbs and garlic can infuse vegetables with irresistible flavors. Roasting veggies, meanwhile, brings out their natural sweetness.

Serving Size: 6

Preparation & Cooking Time: 1 hour and 10 minutes

Ingredients:

- 1 cup red potatoes, peeled and sliced into cubes
- 2 carrots, peeled and sliced into cubes
- 1 parsnip, peeled and sliced into cubes
- 1 turnip, peeled and sliced into cubes
- 1 cup butternut squash, peeled and sliced into cubes
- 4 ½ teaspoons olive oil
- 3 bulbs garlic, cloves peeled
- 3 shallots, sliced
- ¼ teaspoon dried rosemary
- ¼ teaspoon dried thyme
- Salt and pepper to taste

Instructions:

Add the potatoes, carrots, parsnip and squash to a baking pan.

Toss to combine.

In a small bowl, mix the olive oil, garlic, shallots, rosemary, thyme, salt and pepper.

Add this mixture to the baking pan.

Toss to coat the vegetables with the oil mixture.

Bake in the oven at 400 degrees F for 45 minutes or until the vegetables are tender.

36. Butternut Squash Soup

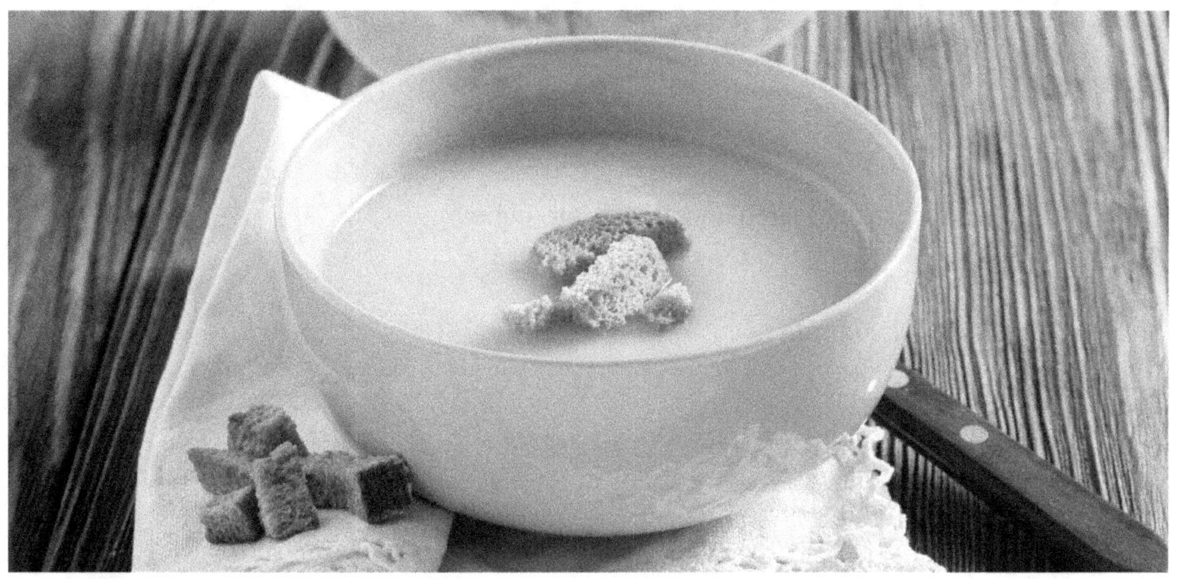

This creamy and filling butternut squash soup can make you feel better when you have terrible symptoms that hamper your day's activities.

Serving Size: 8

Preparation & Cooking Time: 1 hour and 10 minutes

Ingredients:

- 1 bulb garlic, top sliced off
- 1 teaspoon olive oil
- 1 onion, chopped
- 1 sweet potato, peeled and sliced into cubes
- 1 butternut squash, peeled and sliced into cubes
- 2 tablespoons butter
- 14 ½ oz. chicken broth
- 3 ¼ cups water
- 1 teaspoon paprika
- Salt and pepper to taste
- 9 tablespoons blue cheese, crumbled

Instructions:

Preheat your oven to 425 degrees F.

Brush the garlic top with the olive oil and wrap with foil.

Bake in the oven for 30 minutes or until soft.

In a pan over medium heat, cook the onion, sweet potato and squash in butter.

Pour in the chicken broth and water.

Season with the paprika, salt and pepper.

Then, add the garlic to the pan.

Bring to a boil.

Reduce heat and simmer for 20 minutes.

Add the mixture to a blender or food processor.

Process until smooth.

Ladle into soup bowls.

Top with the blue cheese before serving.

37. Root Vegetable Soup

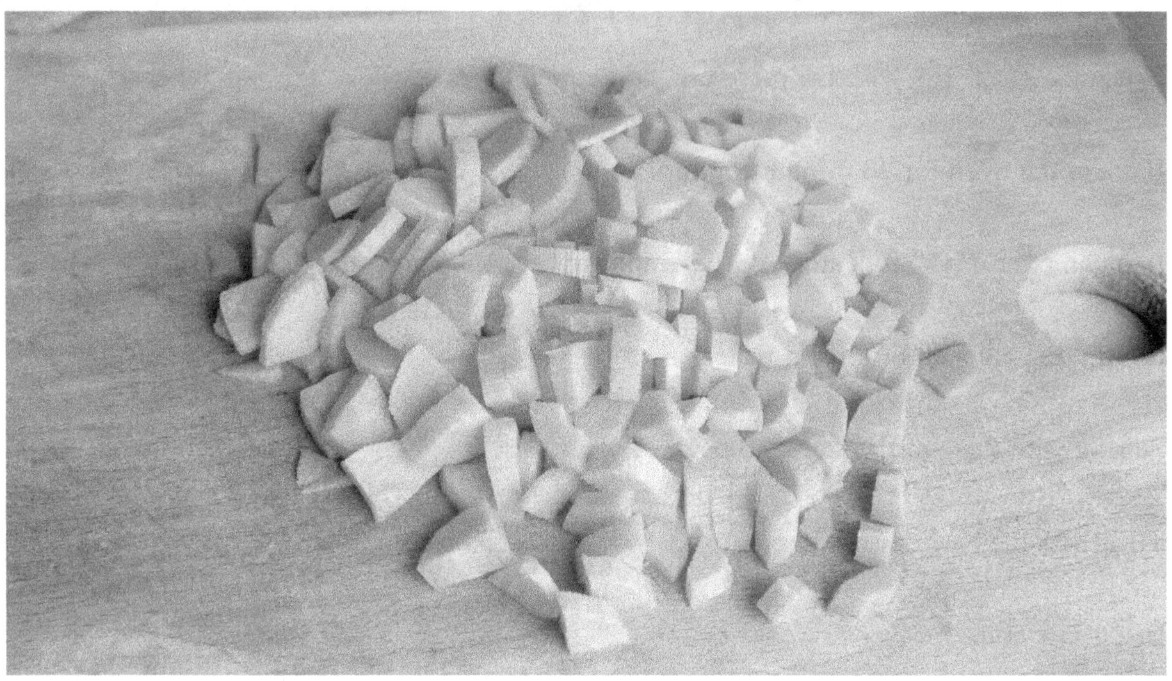

With this root vegetable soup packed with various nutrients, you'll feel better with each spoonful.

Serving Size: 8

Preparation & Cooking Time: 1 hour and 20 minutes

Ingredients:

- 4 strips bacon
- 1 onion, chopped
- 1 green pepper, chopped
- 2 ribs celery, chopped
- 2 leeks, chopped
- 2 carrots, peeled and sliced into cubes
- 2 parsnips, peeled and sliced into cubes
- 1 cup sweet potato, peeled and sliced into cubes
- 2 turnips, peeled and sliced into cubes
- 2 cups shredded hash brown potatoes
- 45.3 oz. chicken broth
- 1 clove garlic, minced
- 2 teaspoons herbes de Provence
- 2 tablespoons fresh parsley, minced
- ½ teaspoon ground coriander
- Pepper to taste
- 1 cup Swiss cheese, shredded
- 1 cup sour cream

Instructions:

Add the bacon to a pan over medium heat.

Cook until crispy.

Transfer the bacon to a plate lined with paper towels.

Crumble into small pieces and set aside.

Add the onion, green pepper, celery and leeks to the same pan.

Cook these in the bacon drippings until tender.

Stir in the carrot, parsnip, sweet potato, turnip and hash brown potatoes.

Cook while stirring for 10 minutes.

Pour in the chicken broth.

Add the garlic, herbes de Provence, parsley, ground coriander and pepper.

Bring to a boil.

Reduce heat and simmer for 20 minutes or until the vegetables are soft.

Next, ladle the soup into serving bowls.

Top with the crumbled bacon, Swiss cheese and sour cream.

38. Melon & Citrus Medley

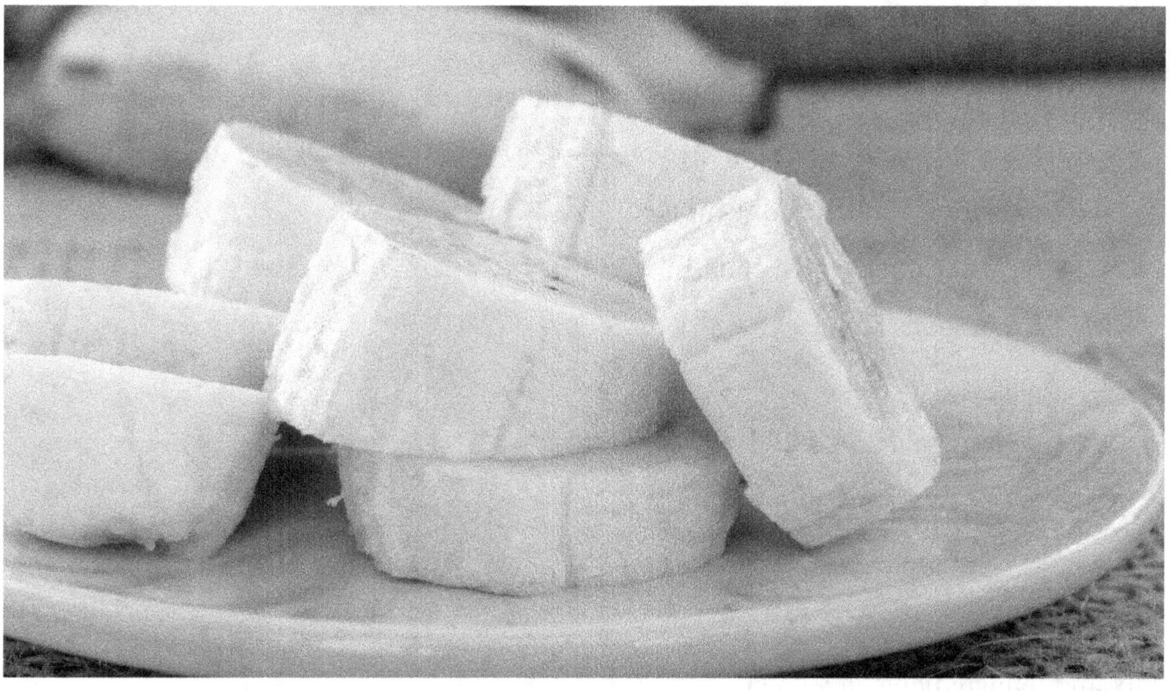

A bowl of refreshing fruits flavored with honey, ginger and mint leaves—this will certainly give you something to look forward on those days when you have stuffed nose or headache.

Serving Size: 8

Preparation & Cooking Time: 20 minutes

Ingredients:

- 2 bananas, sliced
- 1 ½ cups honeydew, peeled and sliced into cubes
- 1 ½ cups cantaloupe, peeled and sliced into cubes
- 2 oranges, peeled and sectioned
- 2 grapefruit, peeled and sectioned
- 8 oz. canned pineapple chunks
- 2 tablespoons honey
- ½ cup orange juice
- 1 tablespoon fresh mint leaves, minced
- 1 teaspoon ginger, minced

Instructions:

Mix all the ingredients in a bowl.

Refrigerate until ready to serve.

39. Carrot Soup with Tarragon & Orange

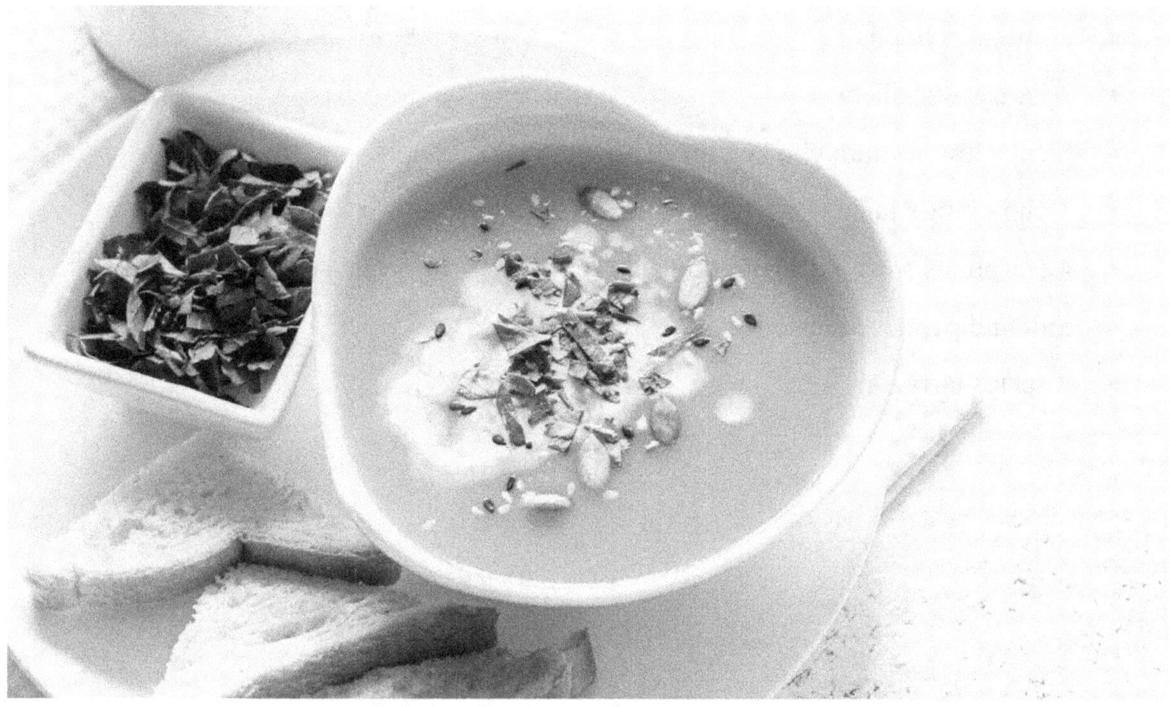

Orange and herbs turn carrot soup into a bowl of potent remedy for flu and colds.

Serving Size: 8

Preparation & Cooking Time: 40 minutes

Ingredients:

- 2 tablespoons butter
- 2 onions, chopped
- 2 lb. carrots, sliced
- 6 cups low sodium chicken broth
- 1 cup orange juice
- 4 teaspoons fresh tarragon, minced
- Salt and pepper to taste
- 8 sprigs tarragon

Instructions:

Add the butter to a pot over medium heat.

Once melted, add the onion and carrots.

Cook while stirring for 9 to 10 minutes or until soft.

Pour in the chicken broth.

Bring to a boil.

Reduce heat and simmer for 10 minutes.

Let cool for 5 to 10 minutes.

Process the soup in a blender or food processor until pureed.

Add the pureed carrots back to the pot.

Stir in the orange juice and tarragon.

Season with the salt and pepper.

Top with the tarragon sprig and serve.

40. Honeydew, Strawberry & Cucumber Salad

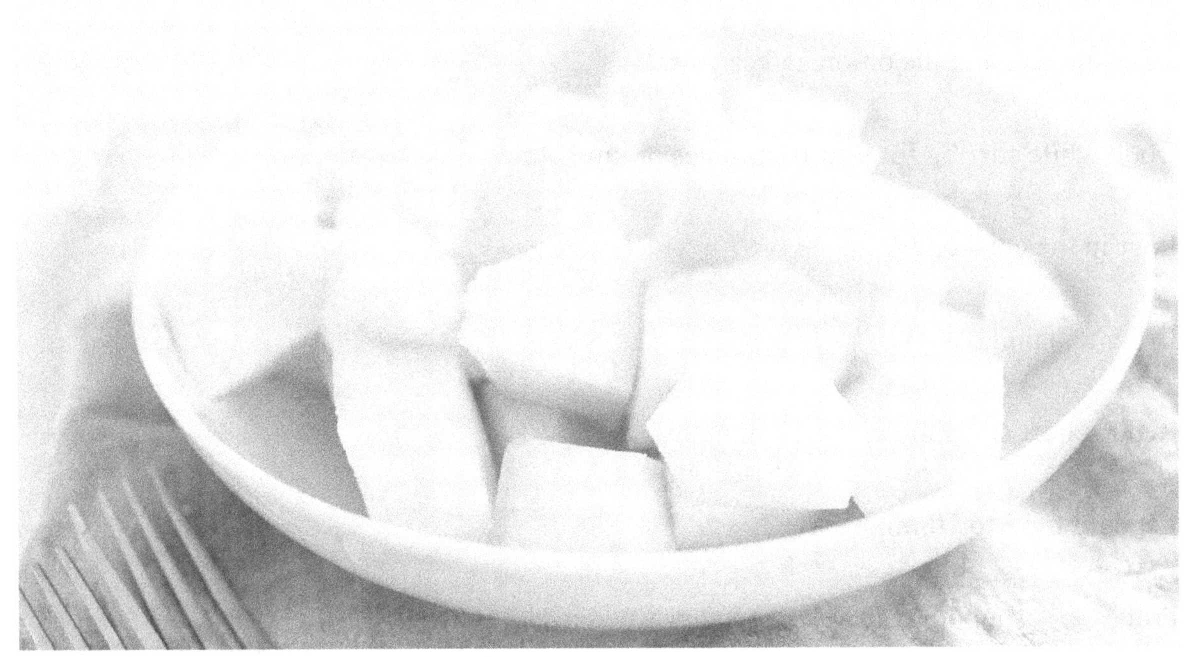

Until you've tried this recipe, you probably didn't know that cucumber and strawberry go well together! You'll certainly enjoy every spoonful.

Serving Size: 8

Preparation & Cooking Time: 1 hour and 20 minutes

Ingredients:

- 1 cup honeydew melon, peeled and sliced into cubes
- 1 cucumber, sliced
- 16 oz. strawberries, sliced in half
- 3 tablespoons honey
- 2 tablespoons lime juice
- 1 teaspoon lime zest

Instructions:

Mix the melon, cucumber and strawberries in a bowl.

Refrigerate for 1 hour.

In another bowl, combine the honey, lime juice and lime zest.

Drizzle the mixture over the fruits before serving.

41. Fruit Salad with Honey & Lime Dressing

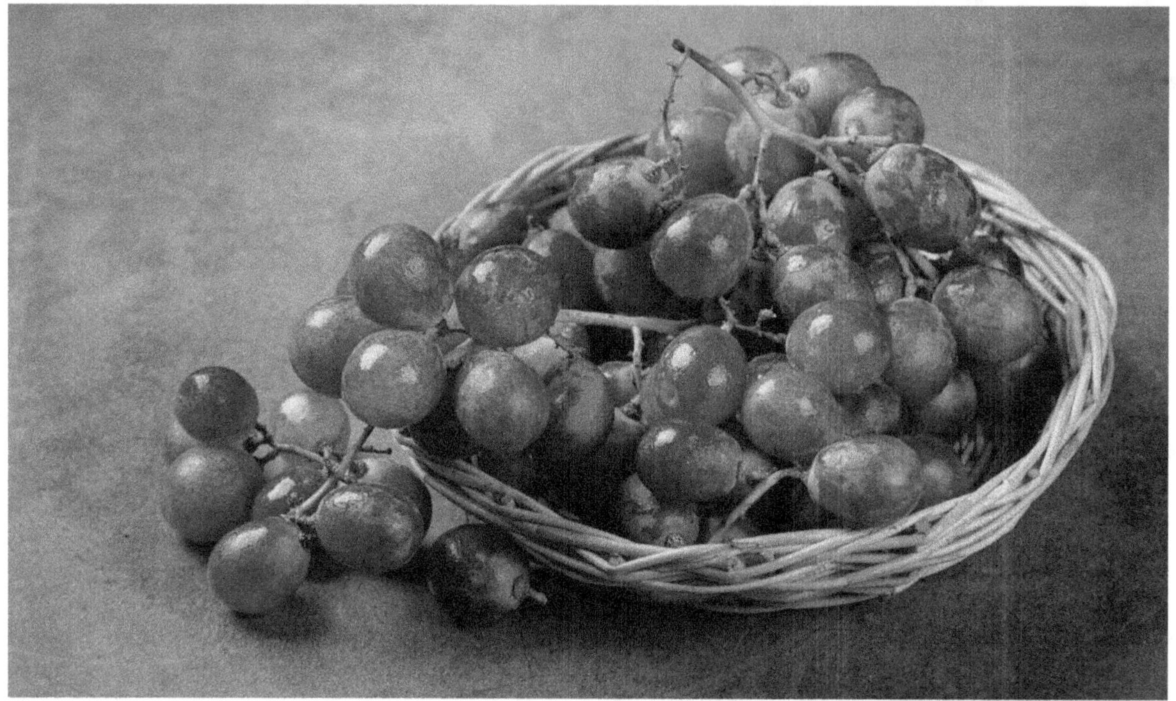

Illnesses like flu and colds can definitely put a damper on your day. But you can fight it off with a bowl of refreshing and nutritious snacks like this fruit salad flavored with honey and lime dressing.

Serving Size: 12

Preparation & Cooking Time: 1 hour and 10 minutes

Ingredients:

- ¼ cup lime juice
- 1 teaspoon cornstarch
- ½ teaspoon poppy seeds
- ¼ cup honey
- 3 apples, sliced into cubes
- 2 cups red grapes
- 2 cups green grapes
- 2 pears, sliced into cubes

Instructions:

Mix the lime juice and cornstarch in a pan over low heat.

Heat through while stirring for 1 minute.

Turn off heat.

Stir in the poppy seeds and honey.

In a serving bowl, toss together the apple, red grapes, green grapes and pears.

Drizzle the fruit salad with the dressing.

Refrigerate for 1 hour before serving.

42. Mashed Cauliflower with Garlic

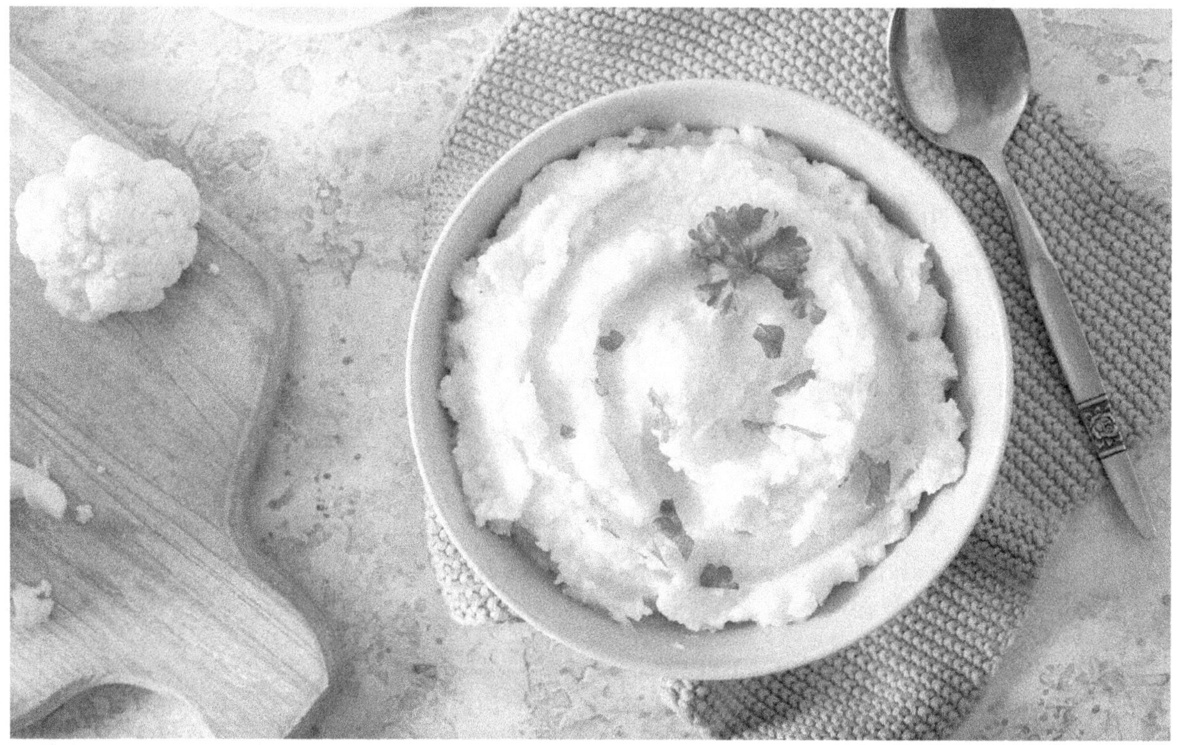

Here's an excellent idea for a quick and simple side dish that also works wonders if you're having flu or cold symptoms—mashed cauliflower flavored with mayo, garlic and chives.

Serving Size: 4

Preparation & Cooking Time: 30 minutes

Ingredients:

- 3 cups water
- 1 clove garlic, sliced thinly
- 5 cups cauliflower florets
- 3 tablespoons low-fat mayonnaise
- 3 tablespoons nonfat milk
- Salt and pepper to taste
- Fresh chives, minced

Instructions:

Pour the water into a pot over medium heat.

Add the garlic and cauliflower.

Bring to a boil.

Reduce heat and simmer for 15 minutes, stirring from time to time.

Transfer the cauliflower and garlic to a plate.

Mash with a potato masher or fork.

Stir in the mayo and milk.

Season with the salt and pepper.

Sprinkle with the fresh chives before serving.

43. Candied Carrots

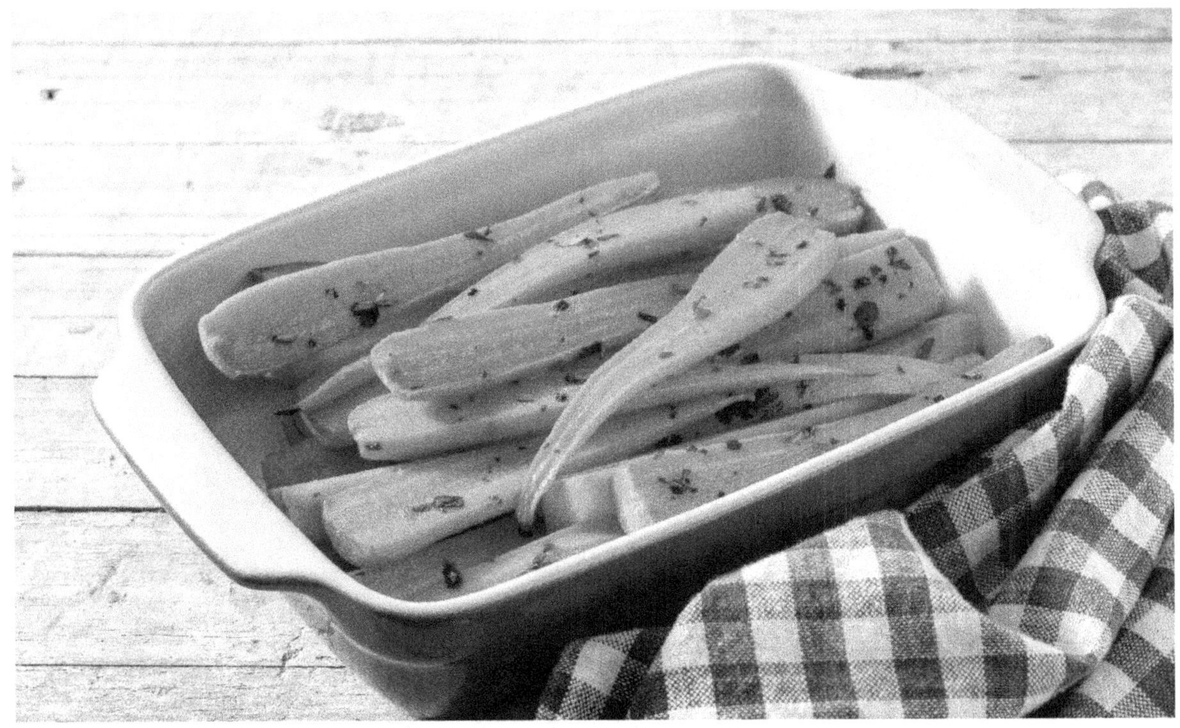

This recipe will easily become your favorite way to prepare carrots. The process is not only easy, but also gives you incredible flavors.

Serving Size: 8

Preparation & Cooking Time: 30 minutes

Ingredients:

- 2 tablespoons butter
- 3 tablespoons brown sugar
- 2/3 cup orange marmalade
- 1 teaspoon vanilla extract
- ½ cup pecans, chopped and toasted
- 2 lb. baby carrots, steamed

Instructions:

Add the butter to a pan over medium low heat.

Stir in the brown sugar and orange marmalade.

Cook while stirring until the mixture has thickened.

Turn off heat.

Stir in the vanilla extract and pecans.

Mix well.

Stir in the carrots.

Toss to coat evenly with the sauce.

Let sit for 5 minutes before serving.

44. Ginger, Lemon & Honey Tonic

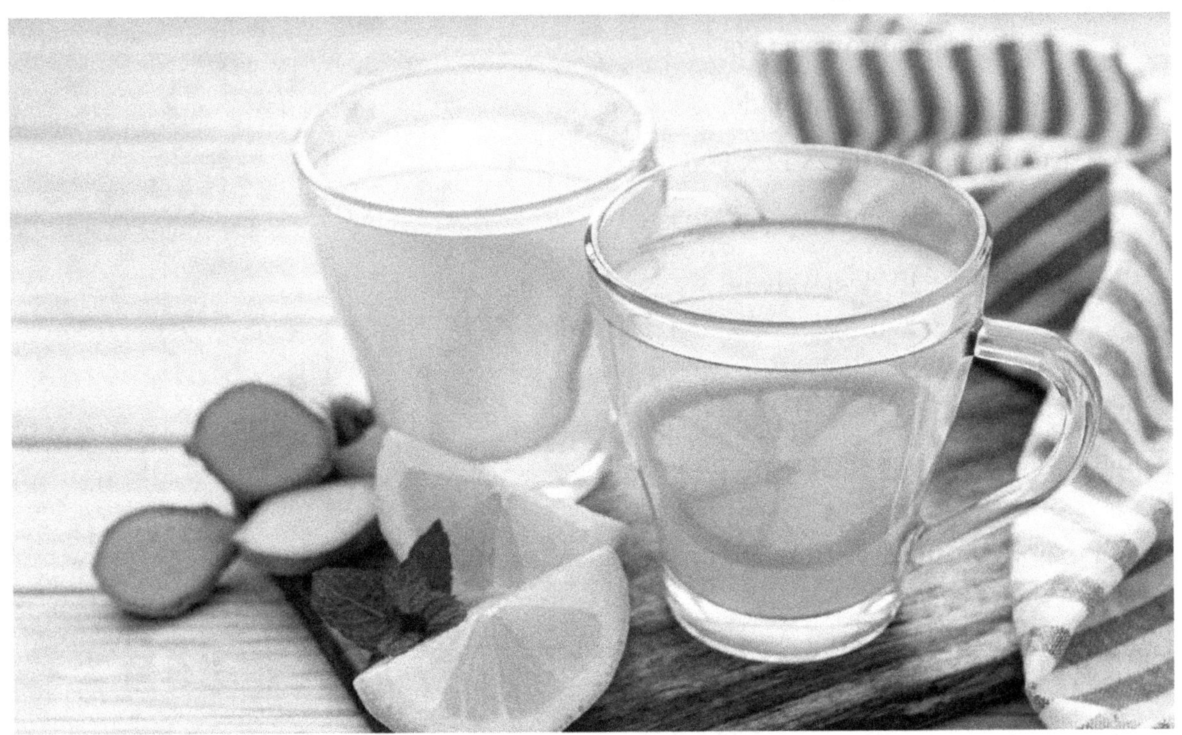

Here's a soothing elixir to calm a runny or stuffed nose and lighten up your mood.

Serving Size: 2

Preparation & Cooking Time: 10 minutes

Ingredients:

- 1 cup water
- ½ lemon, sliced
- 1 tablespoon ginger, chopped
- 1 teaspoon honey

Instructions:

Pour the water into a pot over medium heat.

Add the lemon, ginger and honey.

Heat through for 5 minutes.

Strain the mixture and serve warm.

45. Tortellini Soup with Garlic

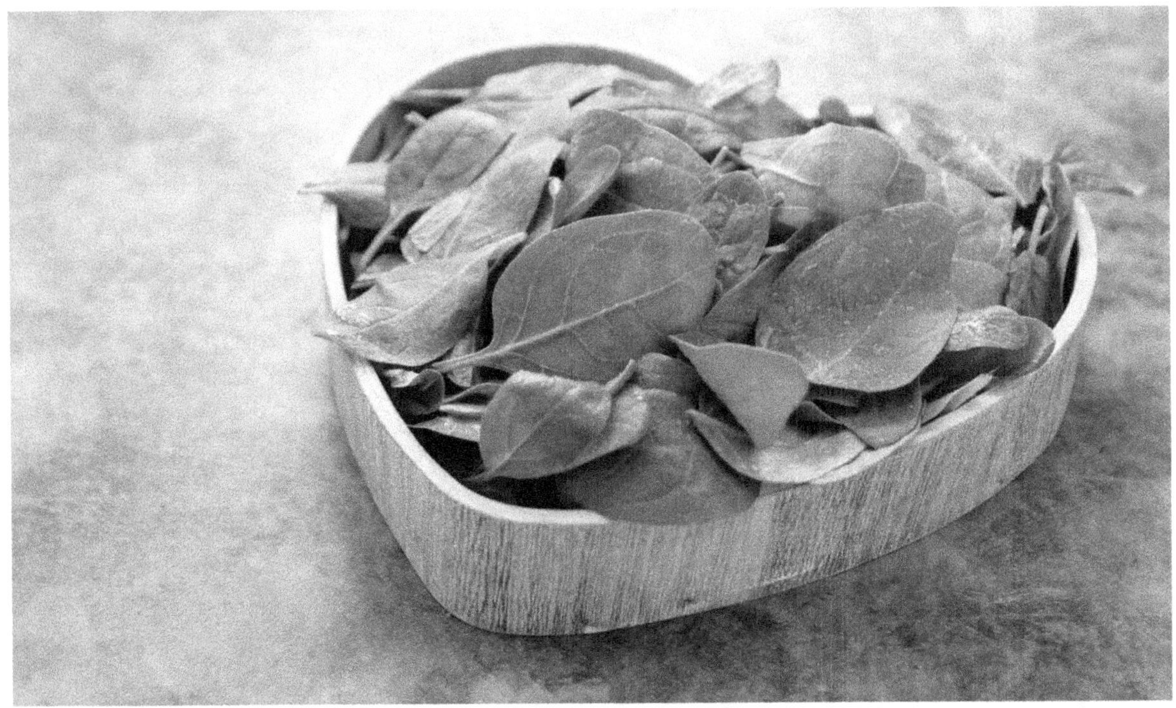

This buttermilk pie crust is an alternative to the traditional pastry crust. Additional ingredients like buttermilk and butter give this pie crust a delicious buttery flavor. To make this recipe extra

Serving Size: 4

Preparation & Cooking Time: 30 minutes

Ingredients:

- 1 tablespoon butter
- 2 cloves garlic, minced
- 45.3 oz. low sodium chicken broth
- 9 oz. tortellini
- 10 oz. spinach, chopped
- 14 ½ oz. canned diced tomatoes

Instructions:

Add the butter to a pan over medium heat.

Cook the garlic for 1 minute, stirring often.

Pour in the chicken broth.

Bring to a boil.

Reduce heat and add the tortellini.

Cook for 8 to 10 minutes.

Stir in the spinach and tomatoes.

Heat through for 3 minutes.

46. Pumpkin Pie Smoothie

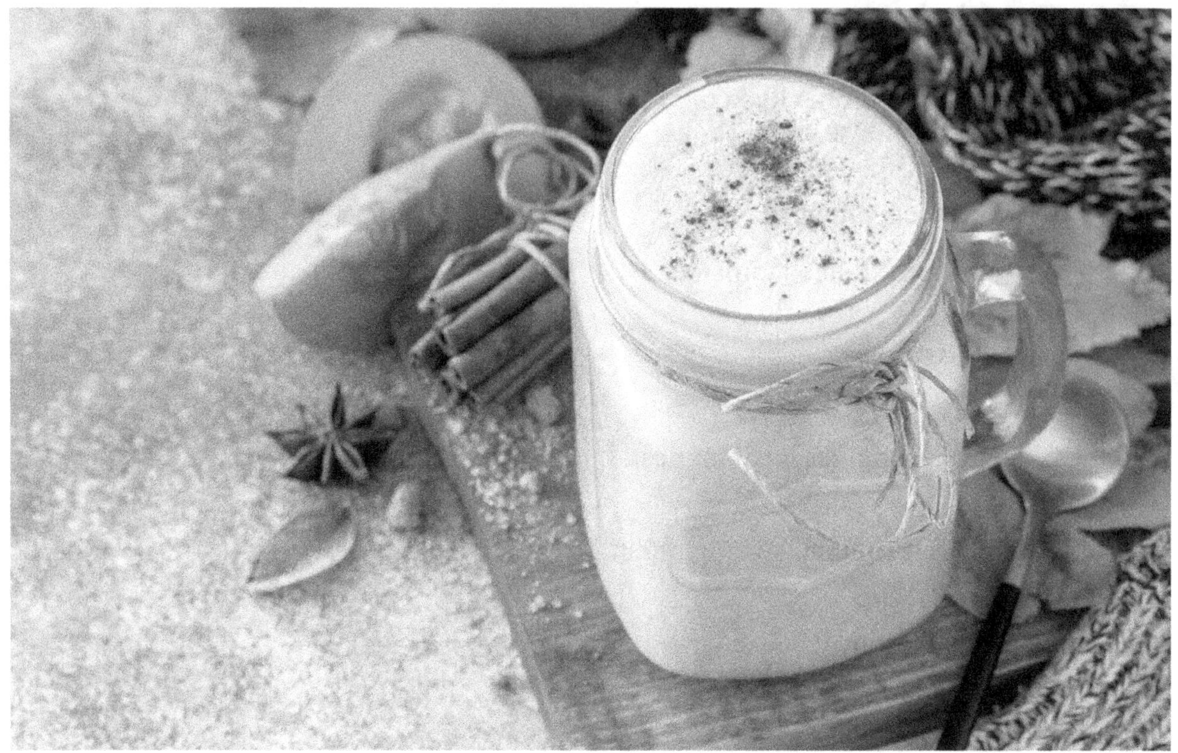

Here's a refreshing smoothie recipe that can surely make you feel better faster. It's made with the same ingredients you use for making delicious pumpkin pie!

Serving Size: 4

Preparation & Cooking Time: 1 hour and 10 minutes

Ingredients:

- 15 oz. pumpkin puree
- 1 banana, sliced
- 1 cup orange juice
- 10 oz. evaporated milk
- 1/3 cup brown sugar
- ¼ teaspoon ground cinnamon
- ½ teaspoon pumpkin pie spice

Instructions:

Add all the ingredients to a blender or food processor.

Process until pureed.

Refrigerate for 1 hour before serving.

47. Honey & Cinnamon Rolls

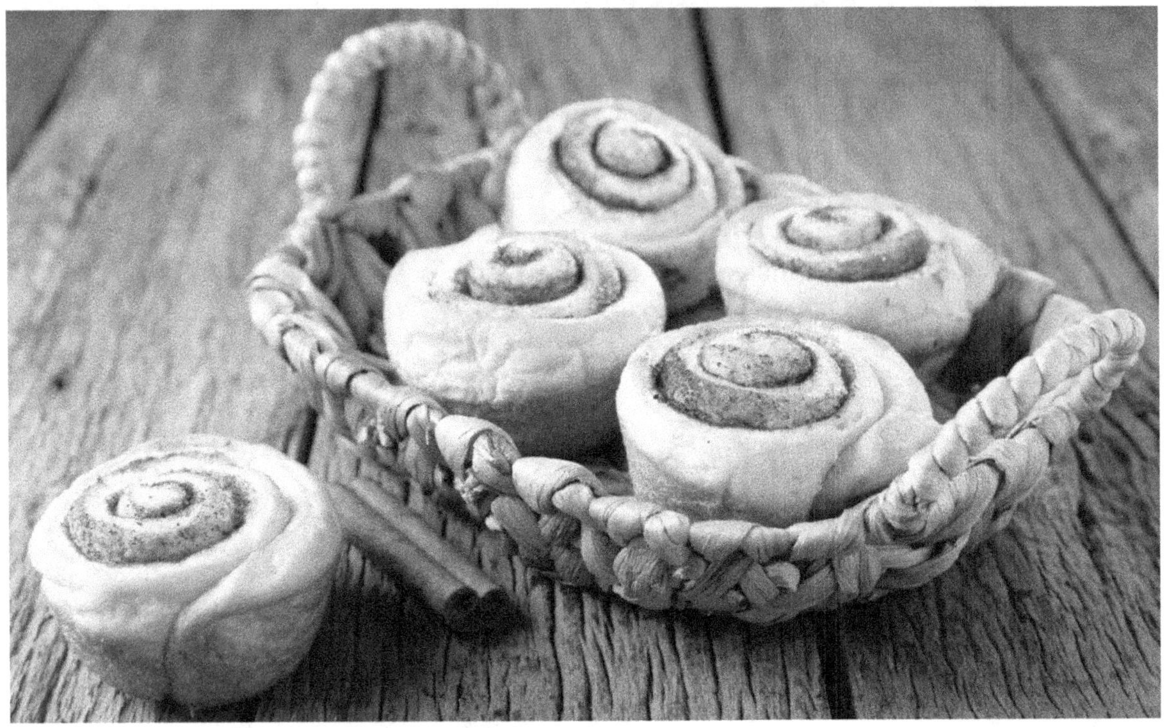

Get relief from flu or colds with these honey and cinnamon rolls. Active components in cinnamon have been proven effective in fighting off various types of infection.

Serving Size: 24

Preparation & Cooking Time: 45 minutes

Ingredients:

- 2 cups walnuts, toasted and crushed
- 2 teaspoons ground cinnamon
- ¼ cup sugar
- 12 sheets phyllo dough
- ½ cup melted butter

Syrup

- ½ cup honey
- 1 tablespoon lemon juice
- ½ cup water
- ½ cup sugar

Instructions:

Preheat your oven to 350 degrees F.

In a bowl, mix the walnuts, ground cinnamon and sugar.

Place the dough sheet on top of a baking sheet.

Brush it with butter.

Place another sheet on top.

Brush it also with butter.

Top with the walnut mixture.

Roll up the sheet.

Repeat with the other sheets.

Bake in the oven for 15 minutes.

In a pan over medium heat, heat all the syrup ingredients until boiling.

Reduce heat and simmer for 5 minutes.

Let cool for 10 minutes.

Drizzle the rolls with the syrup and serve.

48. Lemon Rice Pilaf

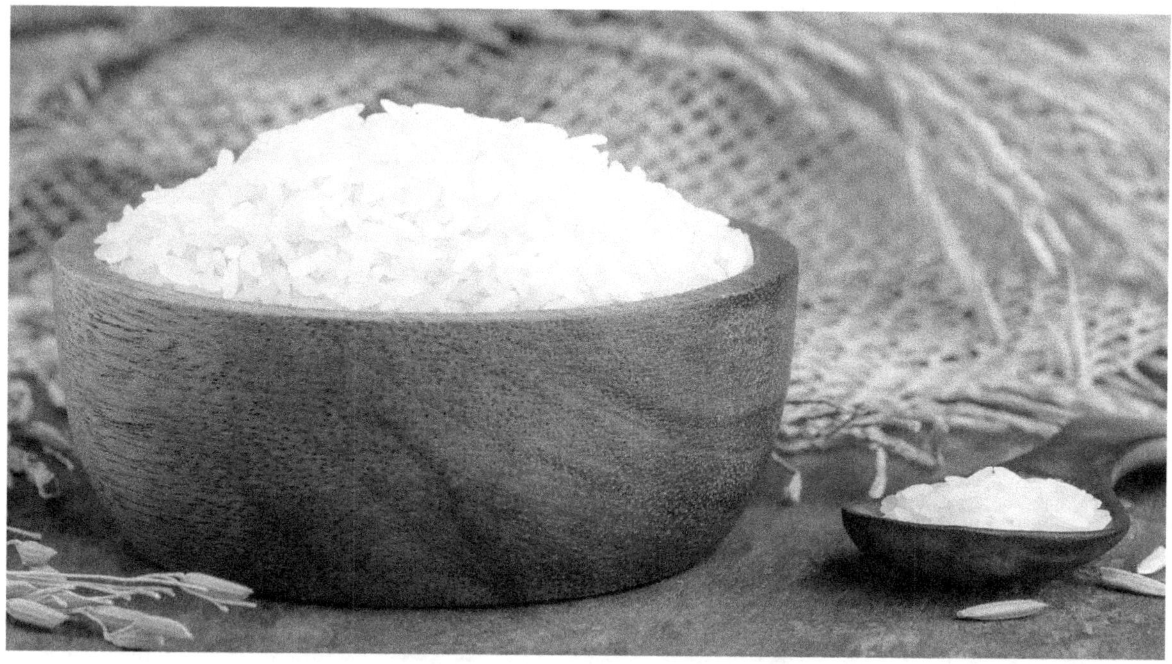

Here's an effortless recipe that you can make even when you're not feeling your best. You'll most likely feel better afterwards.

Serving Size: 6

Preparation & Cooking Time: 20 minutes

Ingredients:

- 1 cup jasmine rice (uncooked)
- 2 tablespoons butter
- 1 cup celery, minced
- 1 cup green onions, minced
- 1 tablespoon lemon zest
- Salt and pepper to taste

Instructions:

Prepare the rice according to the directions in the package.

Add the butter to a pan over medium heat.

Once melted, cook the onion and celery until tender.

Stir in the rice and lemon zest.

Season with salt and pepper.

Heat through for 5 minutes, stirring often.

49. Green Shakshuka

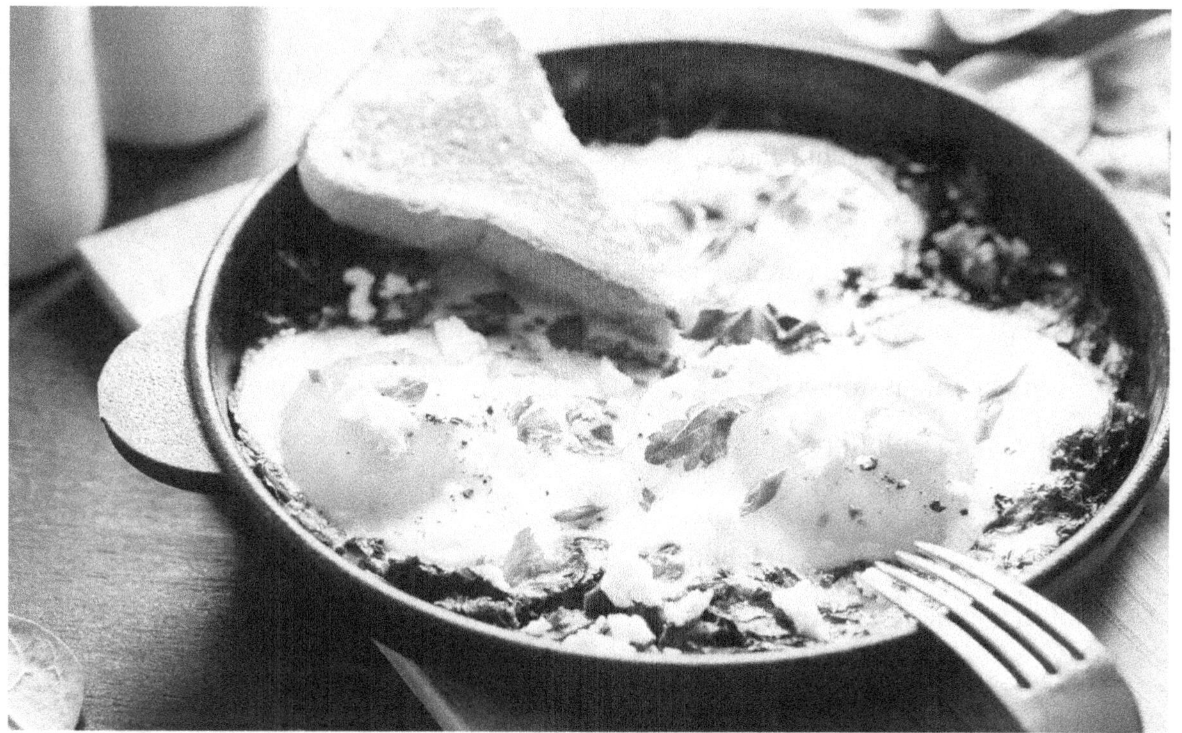

Shakshuka is a traditional Middle Eastern dish made with poached eggs sitting on tomatoes, garlic, onion and olive oil. In this recipe, we make a green version of this dish and pack it with vegetables to help fight off colds or flu. Serve with toasted sourdough bread slices.

Serving Size: 6

Preparation & Cooking Time: 15 minutes

Ingredients:

- 2 tablespoons olive oil
- 1 green bell pepper, diced
- 2 leeks, sliced thinly
- ½ teaspoon dried chili flakes
- 1 teaspoon ground coriander
- 2 teaspoons ground cumin
- 2 cups baby spinach
- 4 green onions, minced
- 2 cups broccoli florets
- 1 cup vegetable broth
- ½ cup fresh mint leaves, chopped
- ½ cup coriander sprigs, chopped
- 4 eggs
- 1 cup plain Greek yogurt
- 1 tablespoon chili garlic paste

Garnish

- Mint leaves

Instructions:

Pour the olive oil into a pan over medium heat.

Add the green bell pepper and leek.

Cook for 5 minutes, stirring often.

Season with the dried chili flakes, ground coriander and ground cumin.

Cook while stirring for 1 minute.

Stir in the baby spinach, green onions and broccoli florets.

Pour in the vegetable broth.

Cover the pan.

Cook for 2 minutes.

Top with the fresh mint leaves and coriander sprigs.

Season with the salt and pepper.

Make indentations in the vegetable mixture.

Crack one egg in each indentation.

Cover the pan.

Cook for 5 minutes or until egg whites are cooked but the yolks are still a little runny.

In a bowl, mix the yogurt and chili paste.

Serve the shakshuka with the yogurt mixture.

Garnish with the fresh mint leaves.

50. Spinach with Garlic & Mushrooms

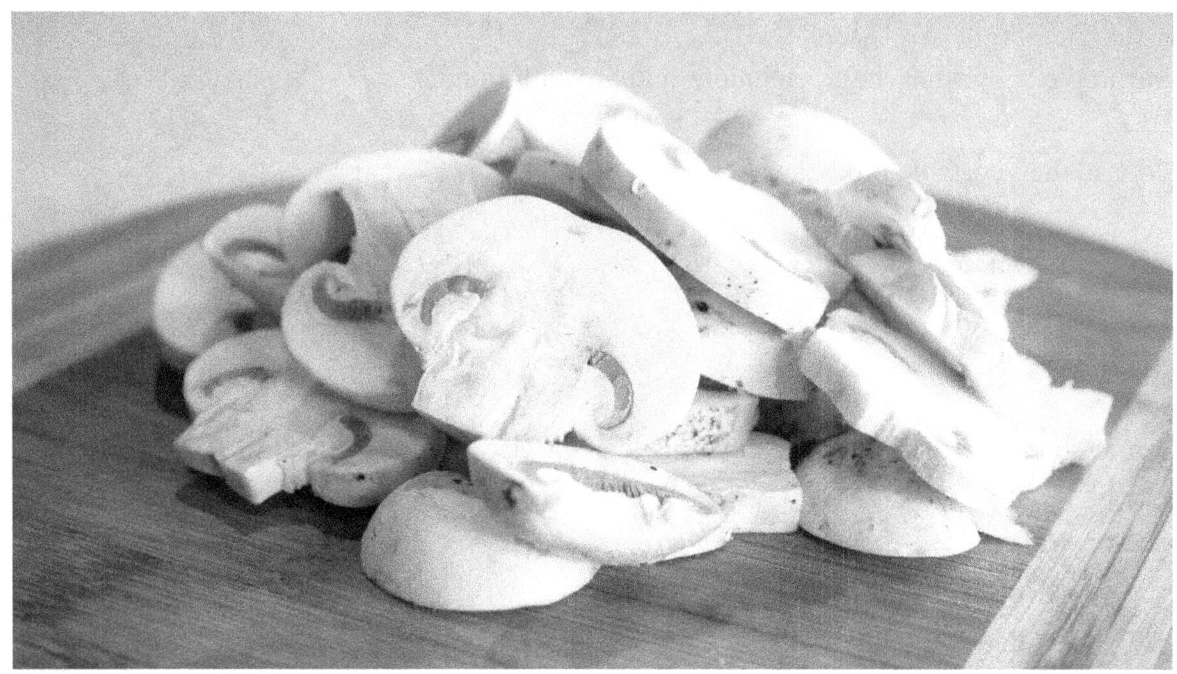

Like other leafy greens, spinach can also your body's immune system and help you fight off flu and colds. Combine it with garlic and mushrooms not only to boost nutrients, but also to enhance flavors.

Serving Size: 4

Preparation & Cooking Time: 30 minutes

Ingredients:

- 3 tablespoons olive oil
- 3 tablespoons butter
- 3 cloves garlic, minced
- 1 cup mushrooms, sliced
- 3 cups baby spinach
- 1 tablespoon parsley
- Salt and pepper to taste

Instructions:

Add the olive oil and butter to a pan over medium heat.

Cook the garlic for 1 minute, stirring often.

Add the baby spinach.

Stir in the parsley.

Season with the salt and pepper.

Cook for 1 to 2 minutes or until the spinach has melted.

Conclusion

With these easy-to-prepare recipes, you'll have no trouble making great meals that are not only flavorful, but are also packed with nutrients that can help ward off your colds or flu.

And soon enough, you'll be back to feeling yourself again.

Of course, you do not have to be ill to enjoy these delightful dishes.

Stay healthy!

Biography

Cooking is second nature to Olivia. This is not a surprise as she comes from a family of chefs. Cooking runs in the Rana family, and it is no wonder that Olivia didn't bother trying to find her root in life.

It was as if her path in life had been preordained for her. She knew that all she wanted to do in life was to be a food expert.

So, after college, she started a small restaurant in her town and launched a culinary school by the side.

Both businesses are doing well, and Olivia has expanded the businesses to a very admirable length.

❀❀❀❀❀❀❀❀❀❀❀❀❀❀❀

Afterword

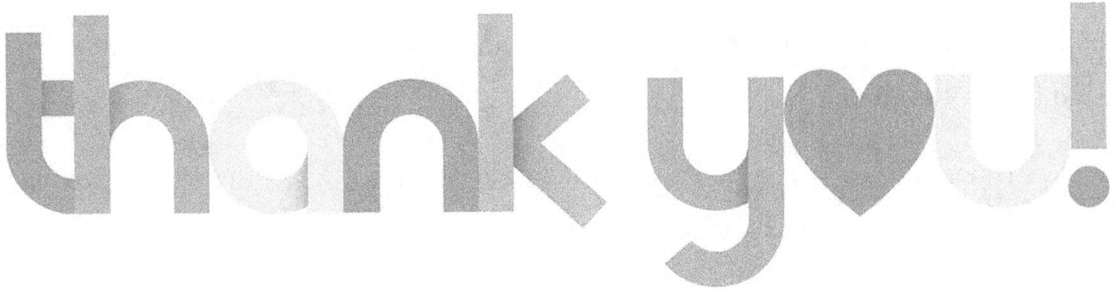

Readers like you are the reason I get up in the morning. I am delighted that you decided to download and read my Books.

I can't thank you enough for choosing healthy living via your choice to engage in healthy and creative cooking. It means a lot to me because I poured my heart and passion into every page of this cookbook. And this is why I hope that you'd get absolute fulfillment from reading and exploring cooking with this recipe book.

I know that there are lots of similar culinary content like this everywhere, but it gives me joy that you chose mine. Hence, I'd appreciate it if you could help with your thoughts about this book. Feedback from customers helps me do better, so I don't mind getting a few from you.

You can do that by leaving a review on Amazon.com.

Thanks!

Olivia Rana